HOW YOUR BRAIN WORKS

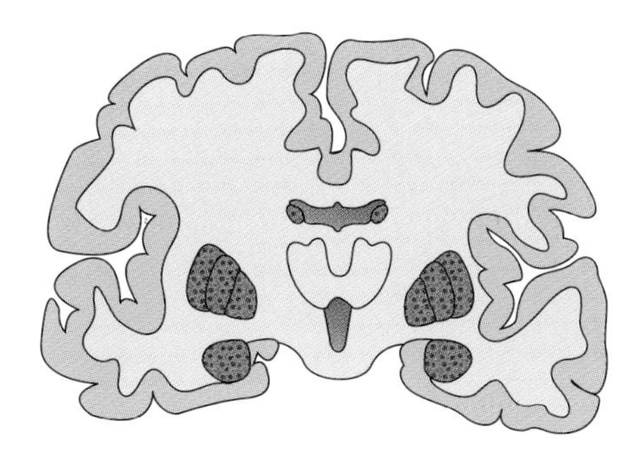

HOW YOUR BRAIN WORKS DESCRIBES THE HUMAN BRAIN IN GENERAL AND DISCUSSES MANY COMMON CONDITIONS AND DISORDERS. IT TRIES TO MAKE YOU A SMARTER CONSUMER OF HEALTH SERVICES AND PRODUCTS, BUT IT DOES NOT OFFER MEDICAL ADVICE AND IS NOT A SUBSTITUTE FOR MEDICAL CARE OR SUPERVISION. CONSULT A PHYSICIAN ABOUT ALL YOUR SPECIFIC HEALTH CONCERNS.

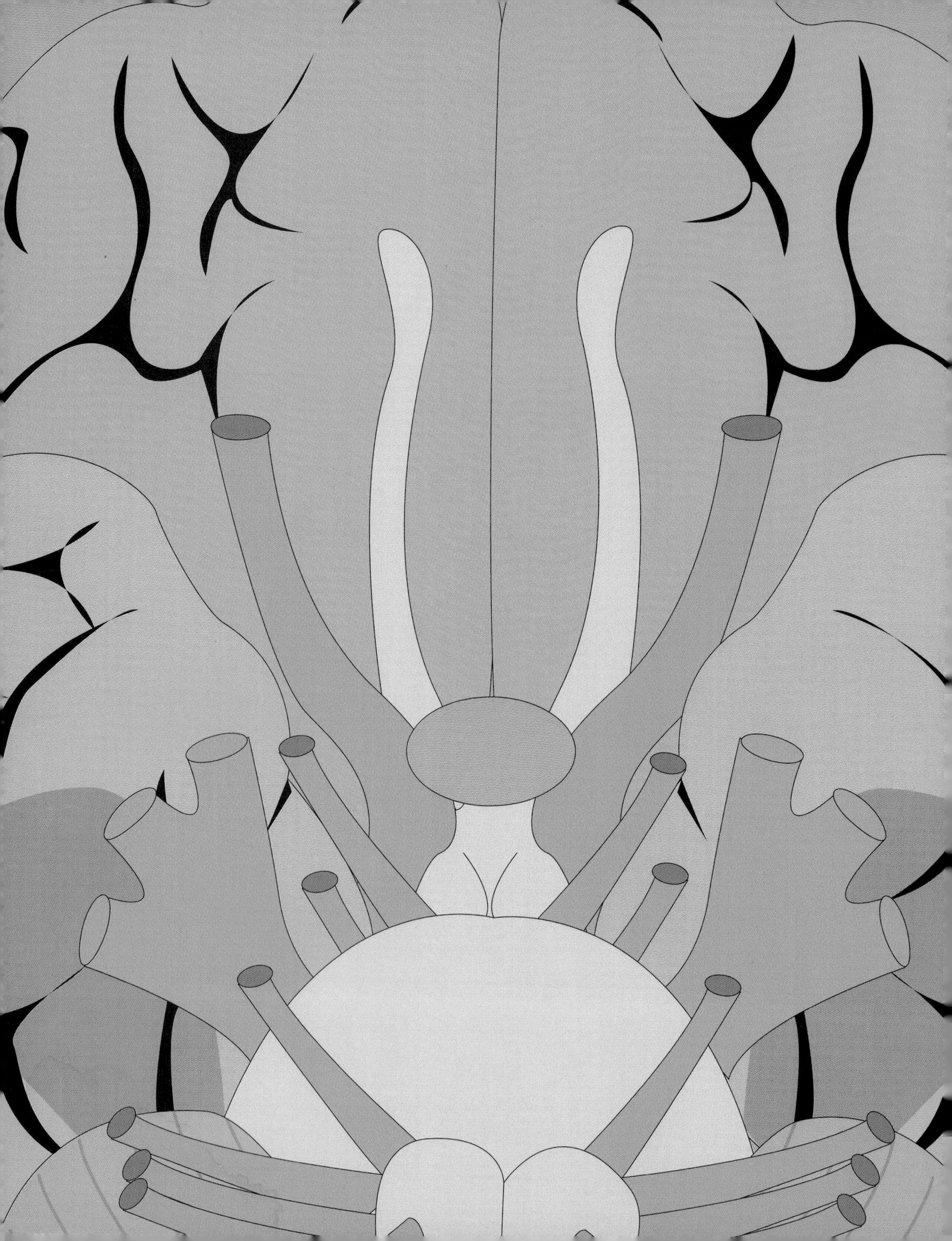

HOW YOUR BRAIN WORKS

ANNE D. NOVITT-MORENO, M.D.

Illustrated by
ERIKA LUIKART

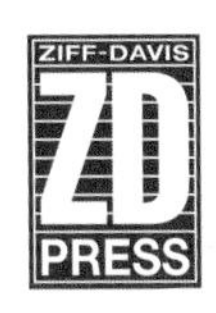

Ziff-Davis Press
Emeryville, California

Development Editor	Mary Johnson
Copy Editor	Kelly Green
Technical Reviewer	Mark A. Young, M.D.
Project Coordinator	Cort Day
Proofreader	Carol Burbo
Cover Illustration	Regan Honda and Erika Luikart
Cover Design	Carrie English
Book Design	Carrie English
Technical Illustration	Erika Luikart
Word Processing	Howard Blechman
Page Layout	Bruce Lundquist
Indexer	Ted Laux

Ziff-Davis Press books are produced on a Macintosh computer system with the following applications: FrameMaker®, Microsoft® Word, QuarkXPress®, Adobe Illustrator®, Adobe Photoshop®, Adobe Streamline™, MacLink®*Plus*, Aldus® FreeHand™, Collage Plus™.

If you have comments or questions or would like to receive a free catalog, call or write:
Ziff-Davis Press
5903 Christie Avenue
Emeryville, CA 94608
1-800-688-0448

PART OF A CONTINUING SERIES

ISBN 1-56276-255-9

Manufactured in the United States of America

♻ This book is printed on paper that contains 50% total recycled fiber of which 20% is de-inked postconsumer fiber.

10 9 8 7 6 5 4 3 2 1

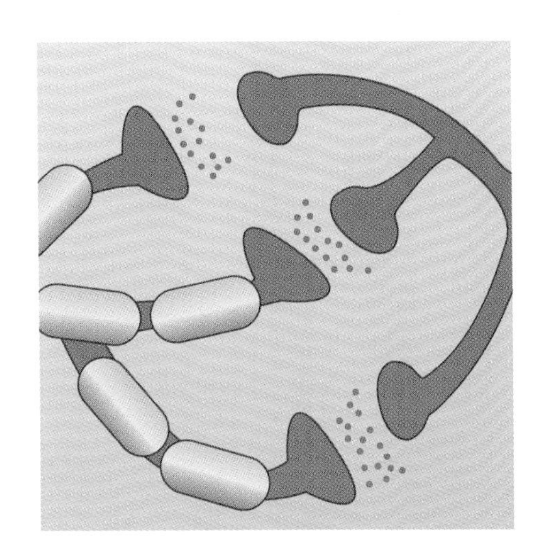

**For my husband, Joe,
and for our children,
Christina, Andrew, and
Michael**

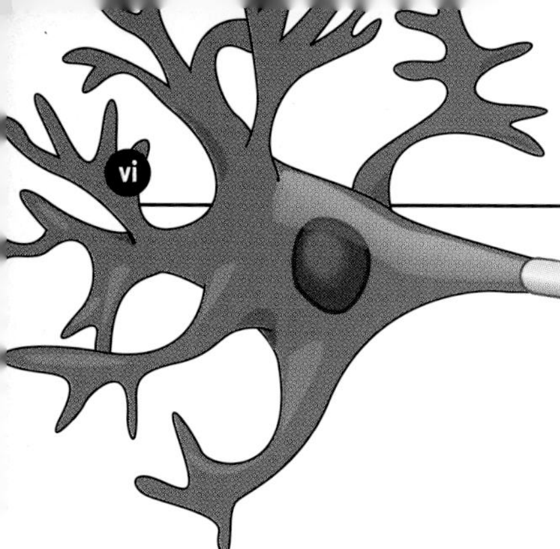

TABLE OF CONTENTS

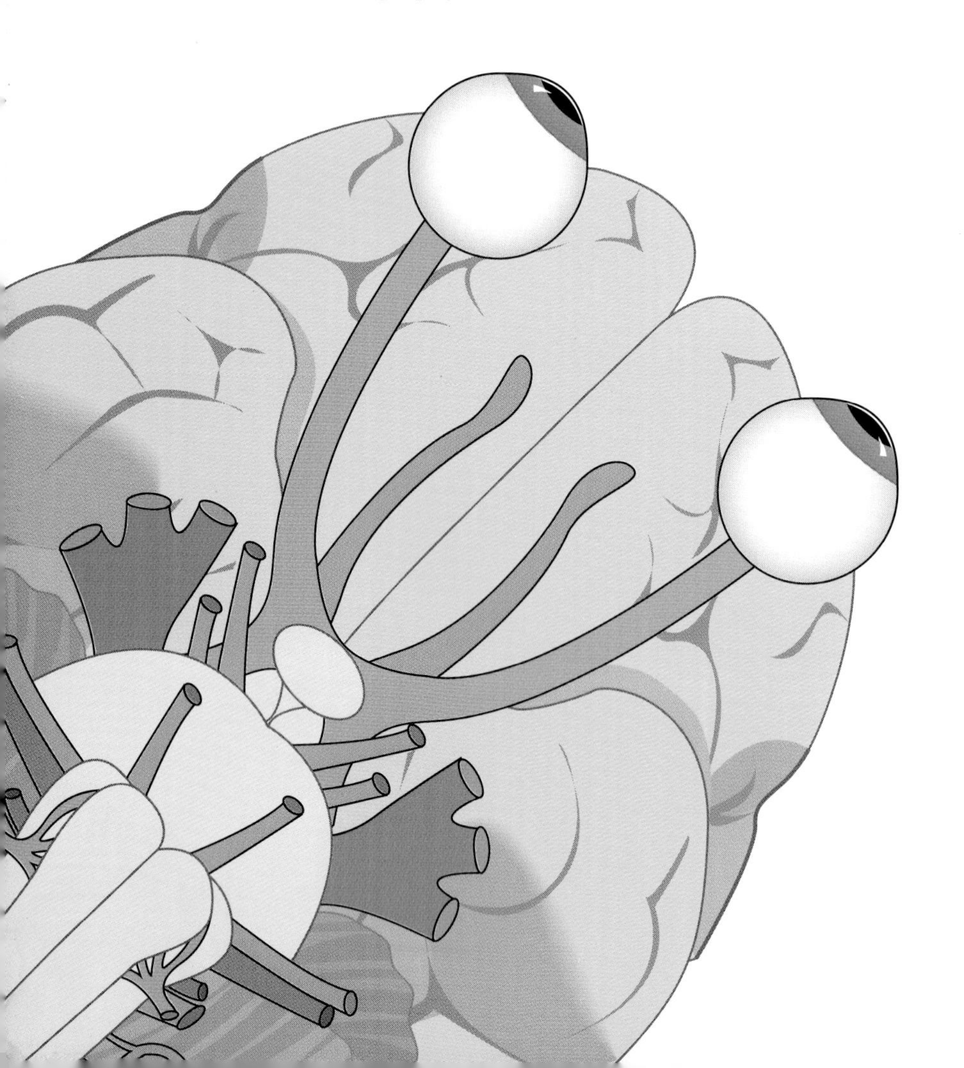

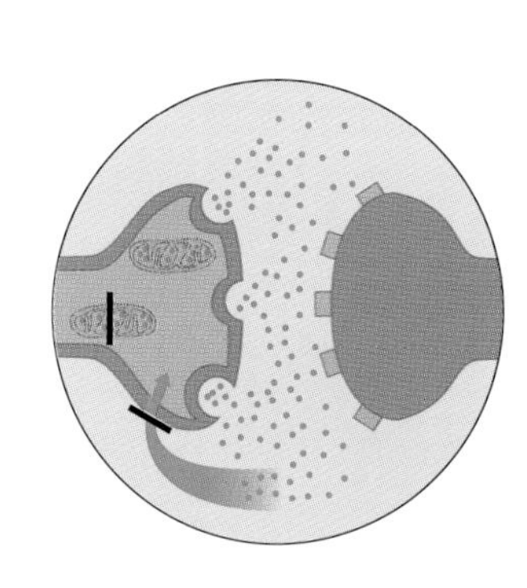

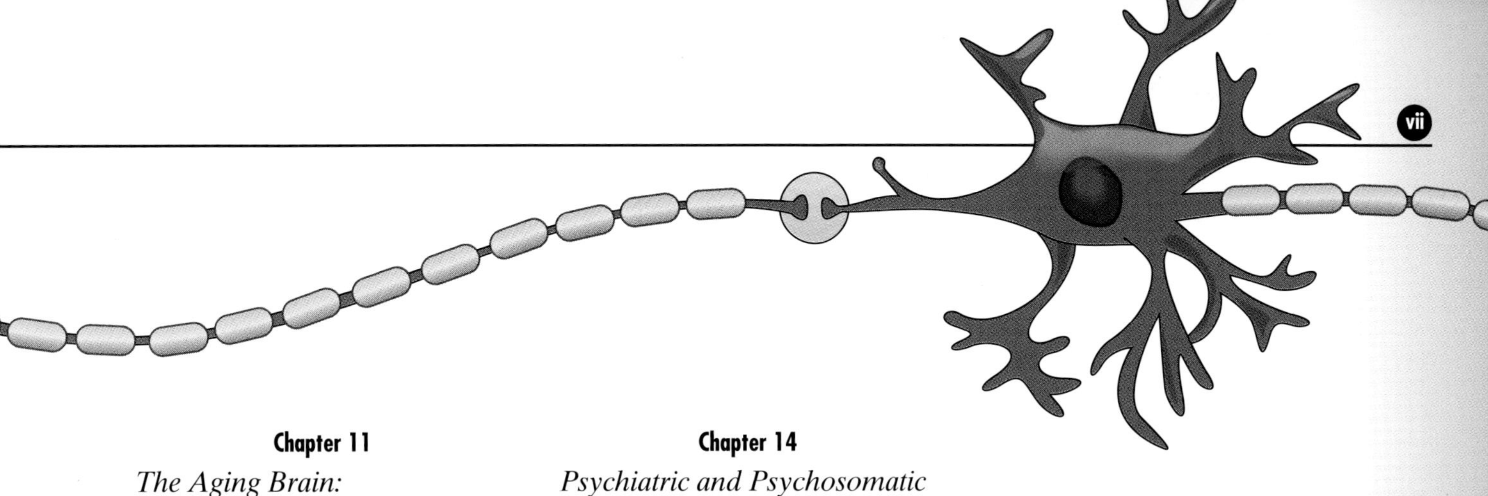

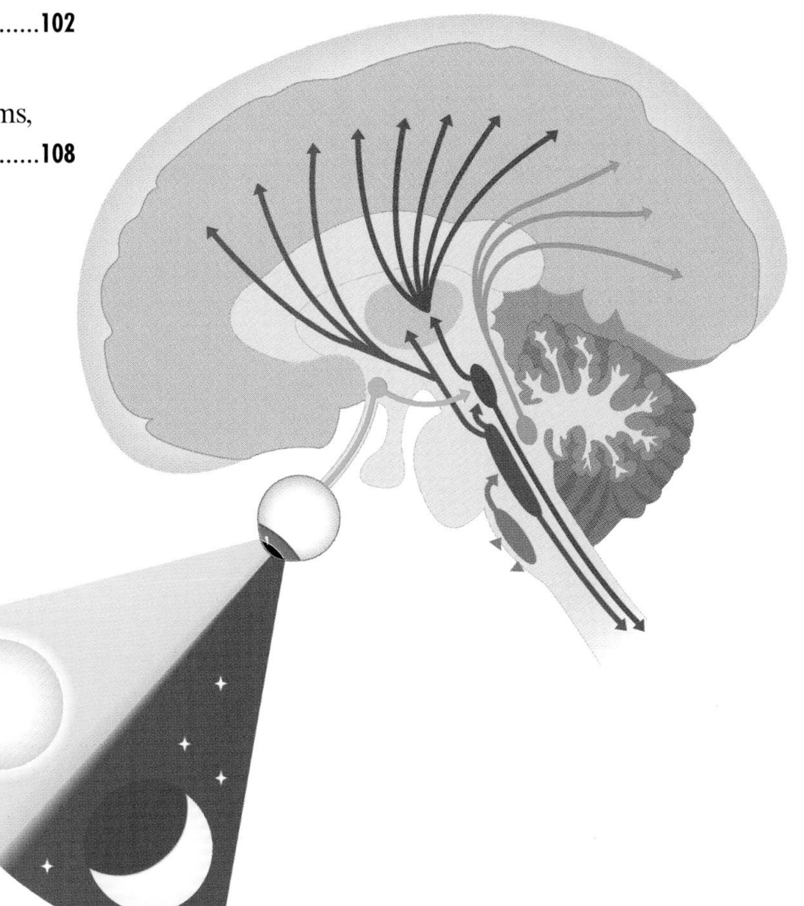

My thanks to all the dedicated, intense, and very professional men and women at Ziff-Davis Press—Cindy Hudson, Eric Stone, Mary Johnson, Cort Day, Kelly Green, Bruce Lundquist, and Howard Blechman. Eric, Mary, and Cort, my sincere appreciation for your confidence in my work and for your most useful suggestions. Special thanks to Mark Young, M.D., for his meticulous technical review.

Erika Luikart, illustrator and visual magician, you turned my Picassos into da Vincis. Thank you for your stunning blend of accuracy and simplicity.

Thanks to the home folks, to my husband Joe (J.G. Moreno, M.D.) for convincing me that an IBM PC is better than an old Royal typewriter, for covering necessary bases, and for sharing my life.

Thanks to my children, who ask hard questions and leave if my explanations run too long—you keep me accurate but brief. Deepest thanks to John and Irene Novitt, to Alice Novitt-Botte, D.M.D., and to Anita Novitt for unfailing support.

A lifetime's gratitude to the talented faculty of St. Peter's College for the Renaissance education of this Jersey girl. Special thanks to Dr. Robert P. Kelly, for teaching me to look for the logic in cellular systems and for encouraging my vocation.

And last, long-overdue thanks to all those patients who have participated in the neurologic and psychiatric studies that have made possible the exploration of the human brain. In times of devastating illness, you have been courageous and selfless. As much as any physician or research scientist, you have been the real heroes in the history of the neural world.

The human brain is history's most unrecognized and underestimated force. It is both the single engineer that has built all of humankind's civilizations and the common source of the errors that have destroyed empires. It has given birth to every single idea of every political and social revolution, directed every act of war, and negotiated every treaty of peace. It has searched for the perfect way to express love and the most efficient way to commit murder. It is the physical origin of human emotion, art, science, medicine, and law. And it is the real physical ark that holds the precepts of every human religion.

Throughout history, the brain has worked to express the spirit of humankind. Because of the brain, the human species, born without wings or fins, has found ways to fly and to explore the sea. Because of the brain, humans have risen above their personal physical limitations as well, so that paralyzed limbs have not paralyzed thought and failing physical sight has not destroyed a clear moral vision. Over and over again throughout the history of humankind, the wonderful, creative, unrelenting human brain has found a way when no way seemed possible. It has consistently turned disaster into new destiny.

After centuries of speculation and scientific exploration, many of the workings of the brain still remain mysteries, even to experts in the fields of physiology and medicine. But these remaining mysteries are no reason for the brain to be avoided or to be seen as a physiologic puzzle that will never be solved. It *is* being solved, little by little, every day. In the meantime, the things that we already know about the brain are intriguing and exciting, and they are not hard to understand.

This book is a combination tour guide, road map, and disaster manual for the human brain. Part 1 begins by taking you on a journey from the outside of the skull to the brain's innermost core, describing structure and function along the way. If you have ever wondered about the brain's major points of interest, you will find them described here. You will discover "hills" that think and feel, nourishing "streams" that flow through underground chasms, and a worldwide cable system that links the entire brain through "electric" communications. You will see how the five senses work, why muscles move, and how the brain controls the heart and lungs. You will search through the brain's emotional core for the places where we feel love and anger, and you will see how the brain controls the levels of body hormones. By the end of Part 1, you will understand where everything is in the brain, what it does, and how that relates to the body as a whole.

In Part 2 you will see how the brain develops before birth, how its landmarks are formed, and how brain cells migrate to the places where they will "live" for a lifetime. You will discover how the brain learns and why it may slowly die without enough mental "exercise." You will also see how the brain ages—what is normal, and what is not.

Part 3 is a short disaster manual where you will learn about some of the most important threats to the brain's safety and security. You will read about the differences between common types of headaches and discover the mechanisms behind both migraine and stroke. You will see how certain forms of epilepsy can recruit wide areas of the brain into dangerous seizure activity, while other forms cause only strange hallucinations. You will learn how tumors threaten the brain from within and how metastases from cancers in other body organs can migrate to attack the brain. You will see why the human immunodeficiency virus (HIV) poses an especially dangerous threat to the brain, and why HIV's actions open the way for many other types of infectious "invaders." You will also see how alcohol and other substances work to directly pollute the brain's environment, and how they may also affect the brain indirectly by damaging other organs. You will discover what is known about the real physical causes of psychiatric illness, and speculate about the possible mechanisms behind psychosomatic diseases.

Last, in Part 4, you will examine what is known about wakefulness and sleep. You will see why eating a large meal makes you feel sleepy and how "sleep factors" related to the immune system may circulate in your blood when you are tired. You will be introduced to sleep science, the study of the stages of sleep and how they affect the entire body, including the heart and skeletal muscles. You will see how one small brain center triggers your dreams and how nightmares may be related to what you eat.

This book was written to be accurate, useful, and easily understood. It requires no prior biology courses or knowledge of natural science. It has no chemical symbols or complicated equations, only simple diagrams with labels and arrows that are no more difficult than a clear road map. If you begin reading it knowing only the front of your head from the back, that's enough. You may finish the book knowing as much as some students of physiology.

As you read, remember to be open to all the possibilities of the brain. Much of it is still frontier territory with undiscovered routes and resources. Your guess may be as good as an expert's.

Take your time. There is nothing overwhelming here. Welcome to the human brain, a finite and rather small world. Only its reach is infinite.

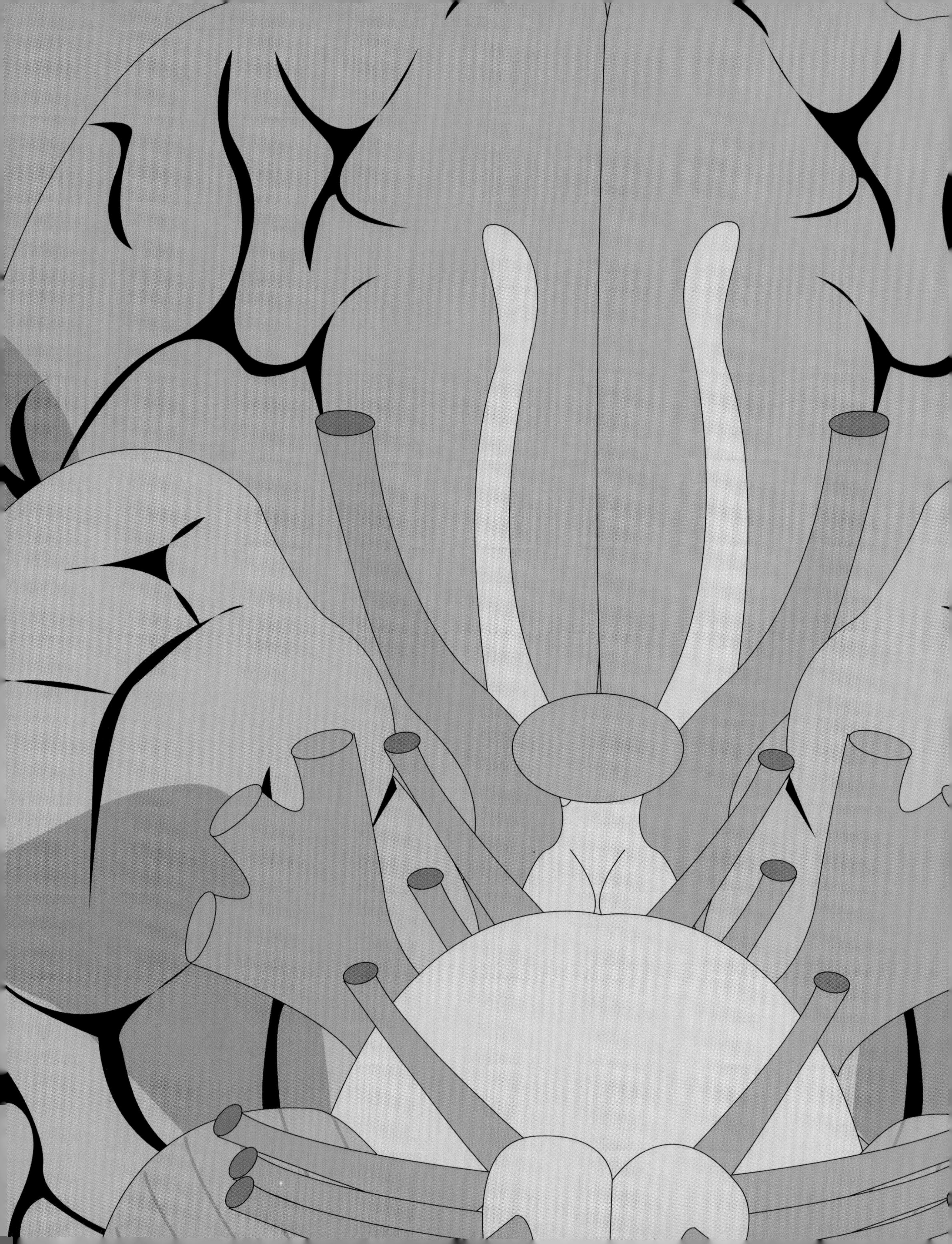

PART 1

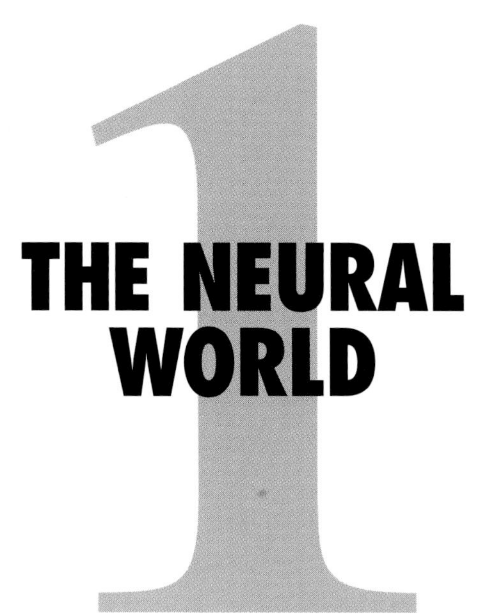

THE NEURAL WORLD

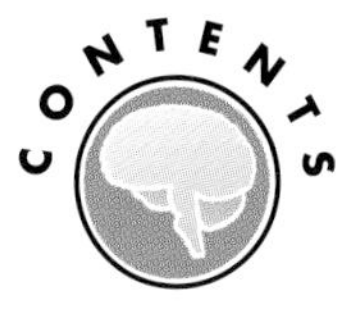

EXPLORATION OF THE living human brain is a rare experience. In many ways, the neural world is as strange and exciting as a distant planet—and definitely more alive. In visiting this world, we will learn as we go: neural geography, culture, language, natural resources, energy requirements, and politics.

But first we have to get there.

Access to the brain is restricted by the imposing barrier of the skull—more than 20 bones, still separate in infancy but fused into one stony vessel by the time we reach adulthood. The major portal of entry is through the *foramen magnum* (Latin for *great hole*), located at the base of the skull at the junction of brain and spinal cord. Alternate routes follow the optic nerves from the eyes, the mandibular nerves from the lower jaw, or the carotid arteries or jugular veins via the front of the neck. Less popular (and much smaller) entrances follow the paths of cranial nerves that link the brain with important structures on the face and neck.

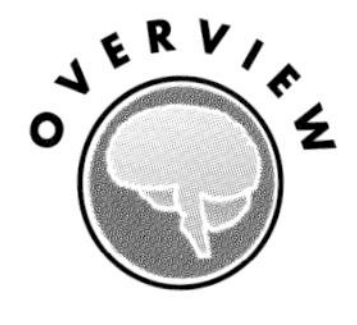

Once we arrive at the surface of the brain, we will need scuba gear. The immediate atmosphere of the brain is liquid cerebrospinal fluid (abbreviated as CSF), which serves as both a nutrient bath and a protective liquid cushion. Above, below, and through the CSF are the meninges, three discrete and distinct membranes that also nourish and protect the brain.

We will first explore the surface of the brain's most familiar geographic feature, the cerebral hemispheres. The twisted surface here is a horror movie cliché, but it serves a useful purpose. The serpentine hills (gyri) and valleys (sulci) provide a way for the brain to grow—by increasing its surface area—in the face of an unyielding container, the skull. The major sulci (called fissures) are the same in all human beings. They form useful dividing lines between the important geographic regions (or lobes) of the cerebral hemispheres—frontal, parietal, temporal, and occipital. Each lobe is the seat of its own set of discrete capabilities: The frontal lobe governs muscle movement, the parietal receives sensory input, the occipital rules sight, and the temporal controls speech. Also centered in the lobes are hundreds of more mysterious capabilities—consciousness, emotions, creativity, illusions. The essence of the "person" is here, too, hidden among the serpentine hills of the cerebral hemispheres.

Below and behind the cerebral hemispheres we find the smaller cerebellum, the balancing center for the brain and the entire body. Under the ridges of the cerebellar surface, body movements are refined and coordinated. When there is poetry in our motions, the poetry is written here.

Moving south, we come to the brain's Antarctica, an area called the lower brainstem. Here two discrete structures—the pons and medulla—form a line that connects the cerebral hemispheres to the spinal cord. Here, too, in the medulla are areas of the brain that can never sleep, because they contain vital centers for breathing and heartbeat control.

Where the medulla ends, the spinal cord begins. The spinal cord is the brain's main communication cable. It brings sensation messages—touch, pain, pressure, hot and cold temperature—from the trunk and extremities to the brain. And in the opposite direction it brings response messages from the brain to the body muscles, telling them to move.

Now that we have a sense of basic brain geography, we can begin to mingle with the neural population. The neural world has billions of living residents. About 10 to 15 billion are neurons—cells that live for excitement. When an excited neuron reaches its threshold, it fires off a nerve impulse—an impressive display of flowing ions and biochemical neurotransmitters. A neuron commits itself totally whenever it fires an impulse—there is no halfway. For a neuron, it is all or nothing.

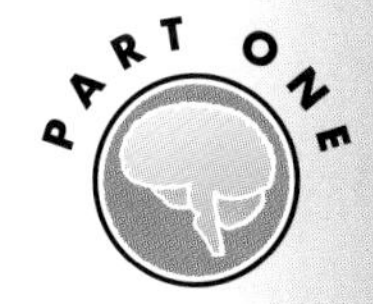

Nerve impulses are the way neurons communicate. Impulses spread from one neuron to another, forming paths and networks of neural excitement. The human body experiences this neural excitement as thoughts, sensations, emotions, and commands for body movements. When a particular pattern of neural excitement is repeated often enough, it becomes faster and easier to duplicate. This is the basis for learning and memory.

Supporting the neurons from nearby is a more sedate population of neural citizens, the neuroglia (or just *glia*, for short). Depending on the part of the brain, the glia may outnumber neurons by five or ten to one. Some, like the star-shaped astrocytes, are very beautiful. All glia are exceptionally industrious, constantly looking after various needs of the neurons and playing a role in brain repair.

Now that we are familiar with the brain's geography and population, we come to a frank discussion of the neural world's political situation. The brain has no natural resources of its own; all its oxygen and energy needs are met by molecules imported from outside sources. Without the heart, lungs, and digestive system—all located far from the brain—the neural world would die.

To meet the needs of its cellular population, the brain exerts neural control over the body's respiration, circulation, and digestion. It allocates one-third of the body's blood supply for its own purposes, although it makes up only about 2% of the body's weight. Sometimes the brain exerts its control through fairly direct means (coughing, vomiting), but sometimes the approach is more diplomatic (loss of appetite, nausea). The brain's medulla is one important center for subconscious—done without thinking—round-the-clock regulation of the heart, lungs, and blood vessels. But some conscious control, such as holding your breath, is also possible.

Body temperature and appetite are controlled through the brain's hypothalamus, a regulatory center located near the pituitary gland, behind the eyes. Growth and reproduction are regulated here, too, via a system of biochemical messengers that act on the pituitary gland.

Some neural activities are intriguing, almost clandestine. We have many more hints and guesses than solid information. What neural mechanisms cause us to enjoy or love? How does stress affect the brain? Can we "decide" not to be sick?

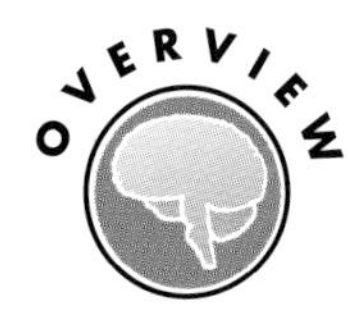

There are so many fantastic issues here. And they all focus on one small fragile world, no heavier than two loaves of bread.

Part I of this book is a guide to the geography and daily life of the neural world. The goal is to make you familiar with the neural environment and its population. The scenery is spectacular, and the natives are *electric*...

Enjoy your exploration!

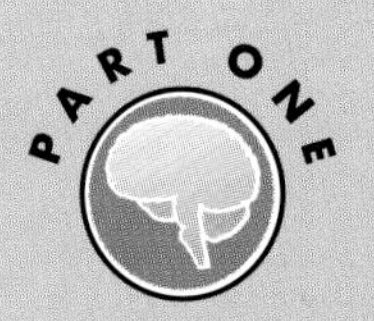
PART ONE

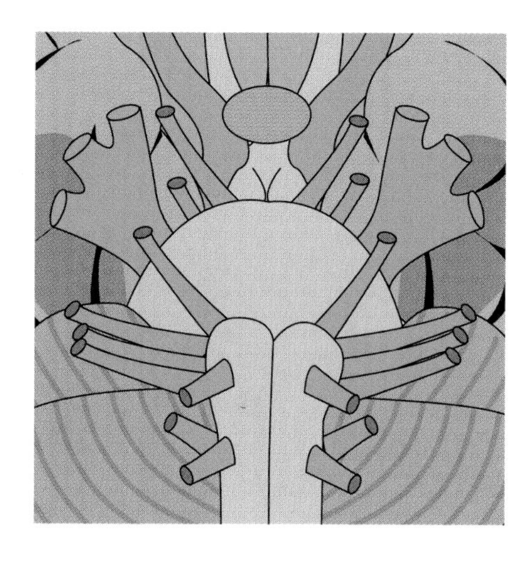

Structure of the Skull and Brain

Neural Geography

THE BRAIN IS NOT an exhibitionist—it doesn't gurgle, groan, or palpitate. The brain is a silent, remote, and armored world whose image, like that of the skull, has been mysterious, even ominous—the subject of horror movies.

When we enter the neural world, we need to forget the Halloween misconceptions and look around with new eyes. The skull is a remarkable vessel, a most definitively human collection of bones. Millennia after death, it still reveals our race, gender, age, and even our diet. At the skull we begin our journey.

The geography of the skull is important because of its spatial relationship to the geography of the brain. The *cerebrum* (the part of the brain responsible for body sensation, muscle movement, and thinking) is divided into right and left cerebral hemispheres, which are partitioned into continent-like regions called lobes. The locations of the frontal, parietal, temporal, and occipital lobes of the cerebral hemispheres roughly correspond to the frontal, parietal, temporal, and occipital bones of the skull.

We will remove the jaw to explore the skull's base, an area that the jaw usually obscures. We will find the *brain stem* (which links the spinal cord with the cerebral hemispheres) and the *cranial nerves* (responsible for multiple functions, facial and visceral). Nearby, we will see the *cerebellum* (which rules balance and coordination) and the pituitary (a gland regulated by the brain).

In the brain, location and function are closely related. Each area of the brain has a specific set of functions—sensation, voluntary movement, coordination, language, or reasoning.

Because of its very specific geography, the brain needs a communications system to link functional areas that must work together (for example, writing requires hand motions coordinated with sight). To accomplish this, the neural world has a network of subterranean cables, the white matter.

Deepest of all, in the brain's innermost core, lies a system of fluid-filled chambers, the *ventricles*. The roof of the ventricles produces cerebrospinal fluid (CSF) that nourishes and cushions the brain. Following the flow of the CSF sends us down narrow passages, through a subterranean aqueduct, and up to the brain's surface again.

In Chapter 2, equipped with a knowledge of the territory, we will begin to mingle with the natives.

Comparison Views of the Skull and Brain

1 Except for the jaw, bones of the adult skull are fused together along jagged suture lines. A frontal view shows three important landmarks: the frontal bone (forehead); left and right parietal bones (upper sides of the head); and left and right temporal bones (lower sides of the head).

Frontal
Parietal (left)
Temporal (left)
Occipital

Frontal
Parietal (right)
Parietal (left)
Temporal (right)
Temporal (left)

2 Shown from the side (lateral) view, a fourth important landmark, the occipital bone, also forms a large part of the base of the skull.

3 Superior views look down from above. The brain's cerebrum (for sensation, movement, and thinking) is divided into two hemispheres, right and left. Each hemisphere is subdivided into lobes. Frontal and parietal lobes are visible here at the top of the head.

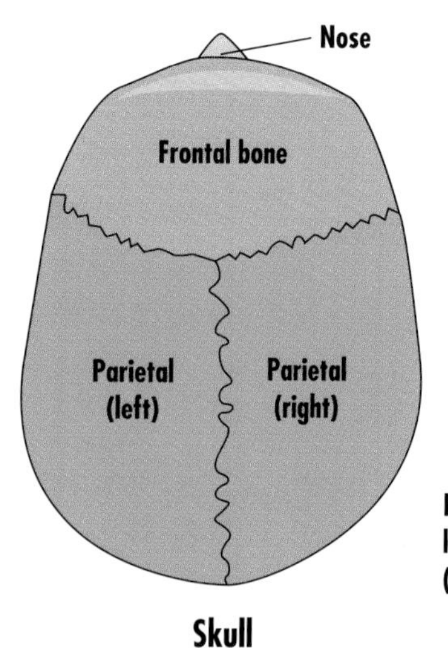

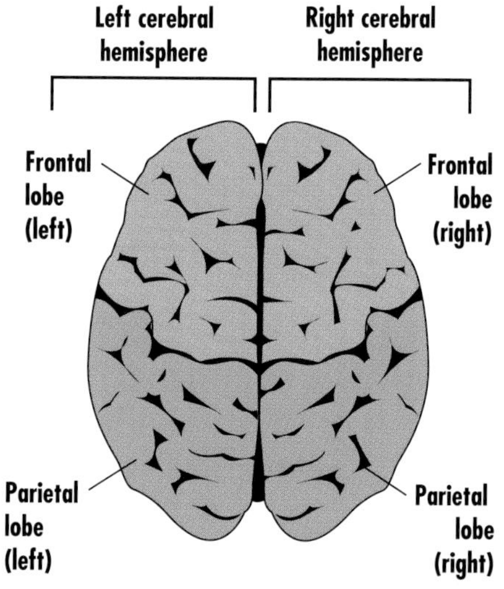

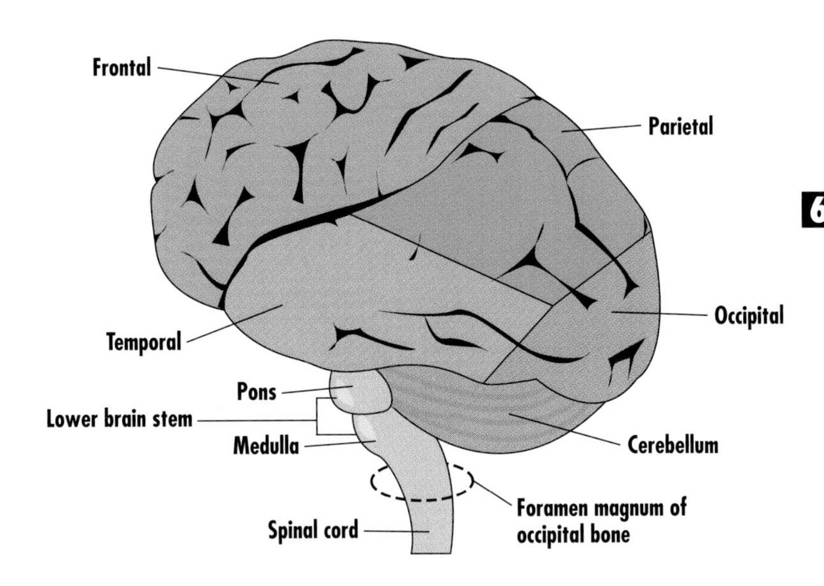

6 Lateral views show a geographic summary of the skull and brain. The average adult brain weighs about 1,400 grams (45 ounces). Larger brains do not necessarily mean greater intelligence.

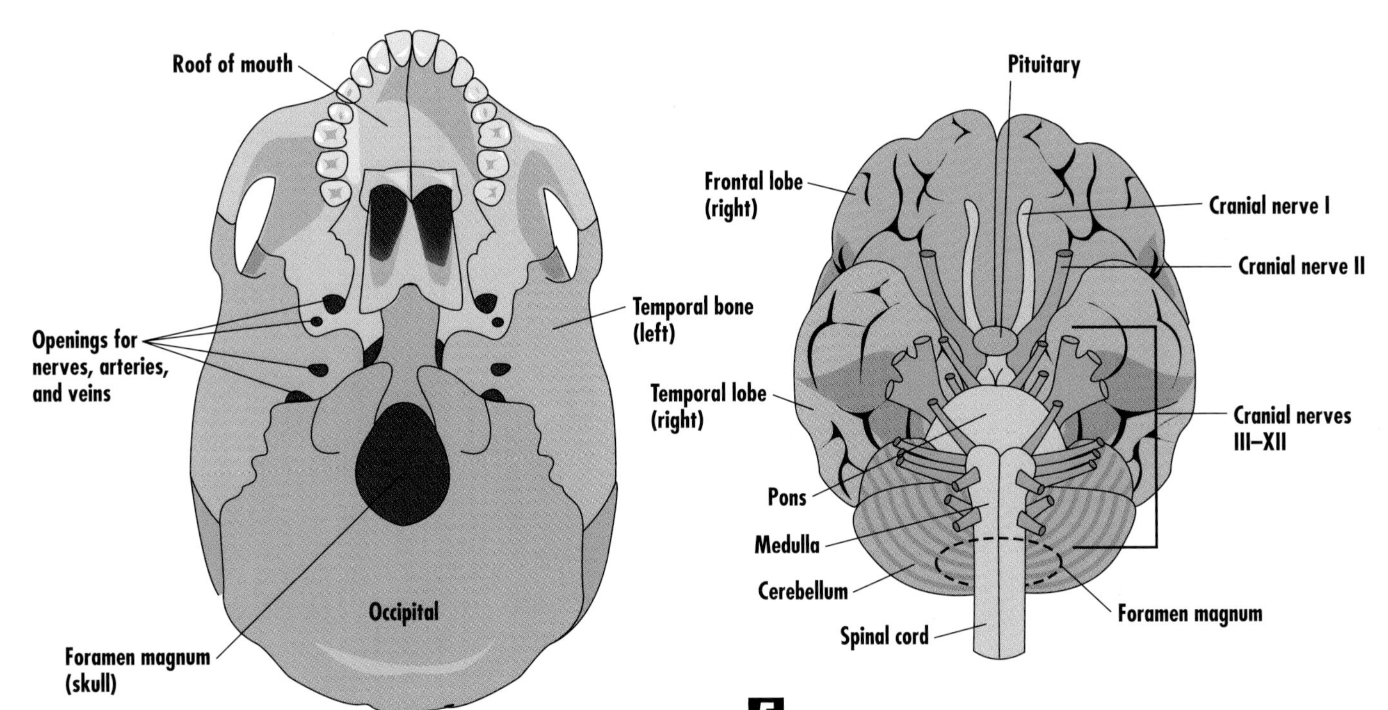

(View from base of skull looking up)

4 A rare perspective shows the base of the skull with the jaw removed. The occipital bone has the *foramen magnum*, the largest opening into the brain, which marks the junction between brain and spinal cord. Smaller skull openings are passages for the carotid arteries, jugular veins, and cranial nerves.

5 The corresponding view of the base of the brain allows us to see portions of the frontal and temporal lobes of the cerebral hemispheres, the cerebellum (for balance and coordination), the medulla (which connects the brain and spinal cord and controls vital functions), the pons (an important relay center), and the 12 cranial nerves. The pituitary gland is shown in close relationship to the brain.

Mountains and Valleys

1 A *gyrus* (plural, gyri) is a hill on the brain's surface, and a *sulcus* (plural, sulci) is a valley. A *fissure* is a very deep sulcus. The longitudinal fissure divides the brain into left and right hemispheres, or sides. Many brain functions (such as sensation and voluntary movement) are *contralateral* (opposite sided), which means that the left side of the brain controls the right side of the body, and vice versa. The central sulcus separates the frontal from the parietal lobes.

2 Each *frontal lobe* controls voluntary movements on the contralateral (opposite) side of the body. Frontal lobes also influence the planning of movement and receive the sense of smell. In 99% of right-handed people and 60% of left-handed people, the left hemisphere is *dominant* (that is, it controls language), with the left frontal lobe in control of verbal expression. In people with a dominant right hemisphere, the right frontal lobe controls verbal expression.

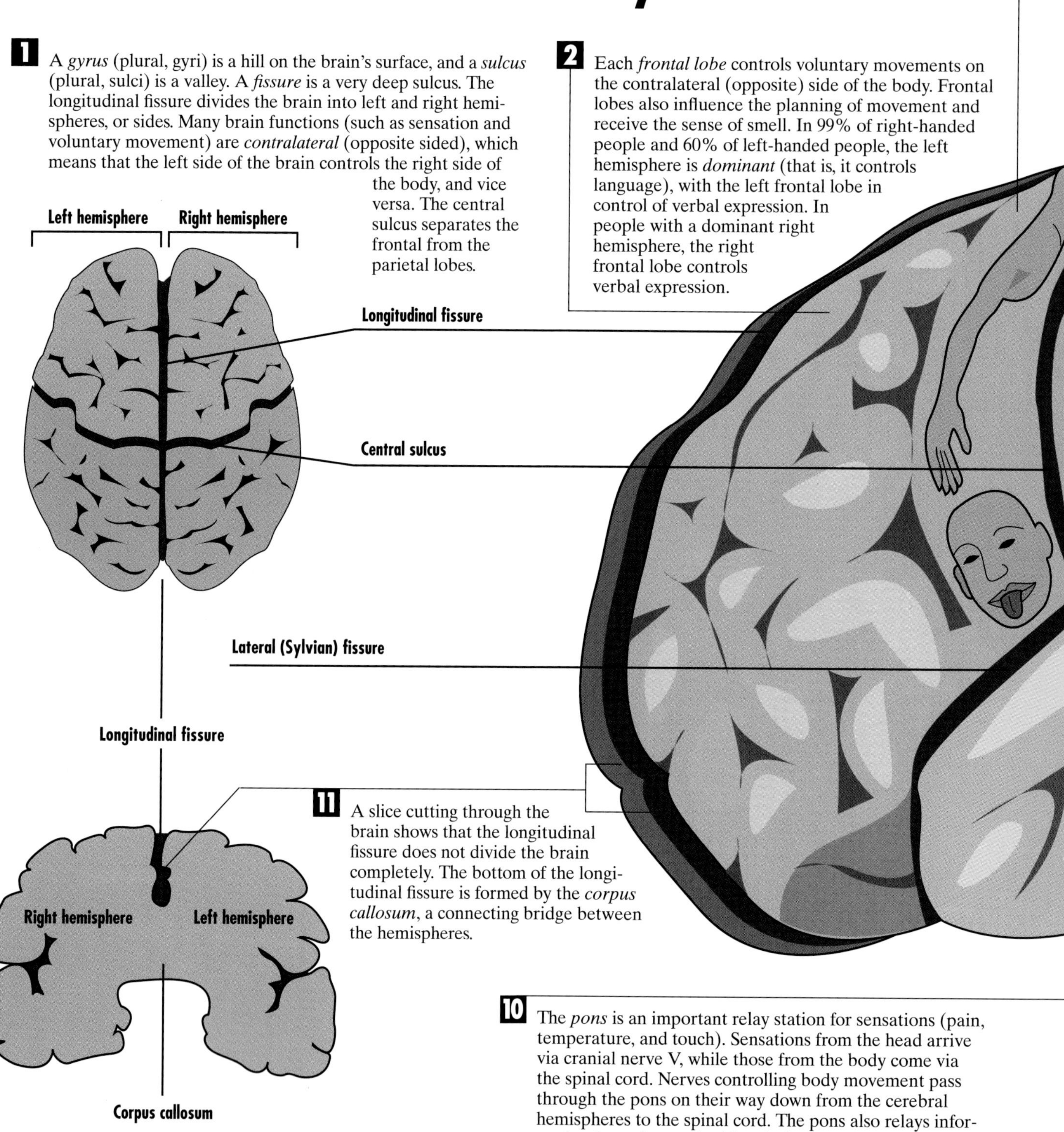

11 A slice cutting through the brain shows that the longitudinal fissure does not divide the brain completely. The bottom of the longitudinal fissure is formed by the *corpus callosum*, a connecting bridge between the hemispheres.

10 The *pons* is an important relay station for sensations (pain, temperature, and touch). Sensations from the head arrive via cranial nerve V, while those from the body come via the spinal cord. Nerves controlling body movement pass through the pons on their way down from the cerebral hemispheres to the spinal cord. The pons also relays information from the cerebral hemispheres to the cerebellum.

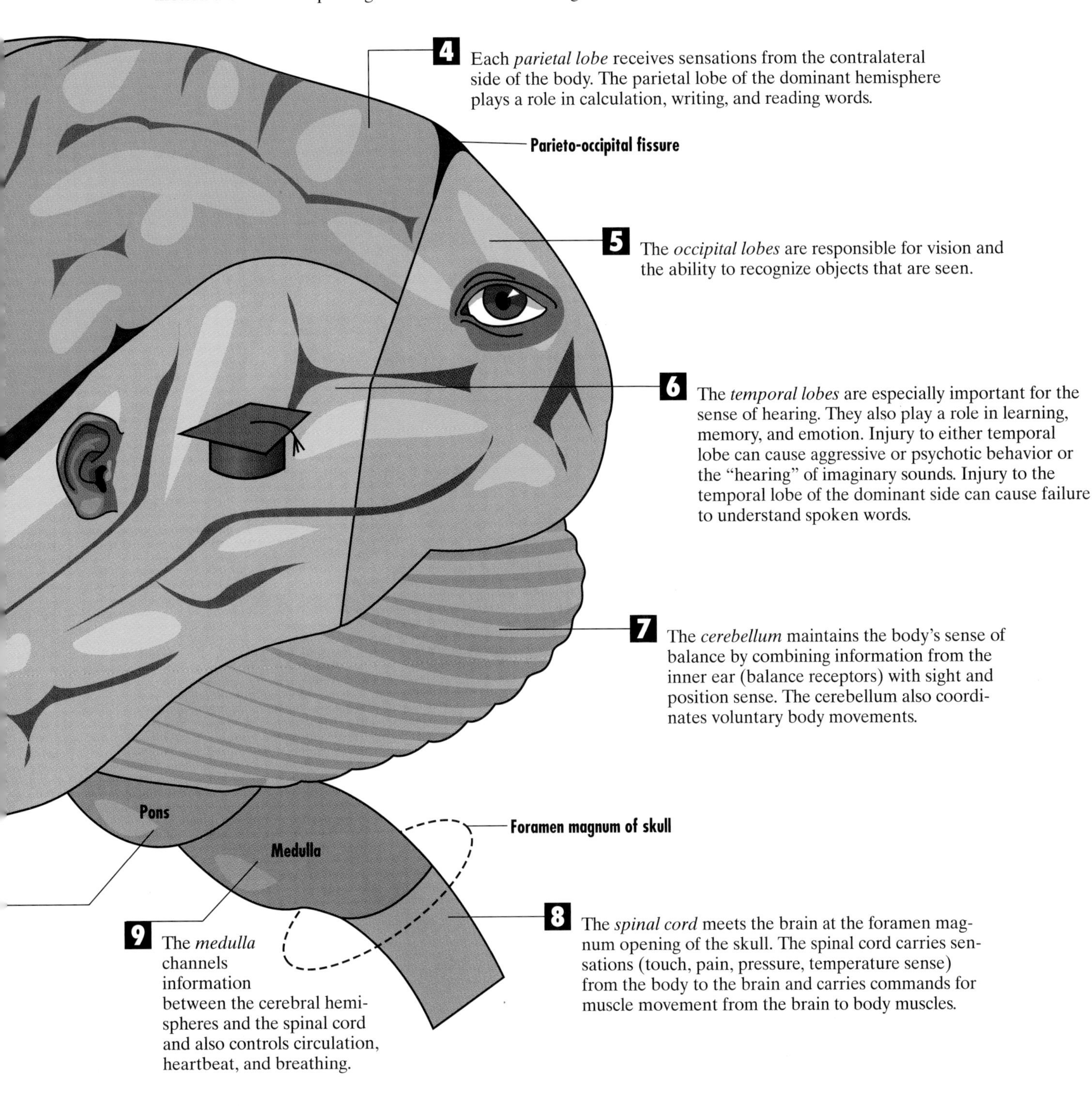

3 The *precentral gyrus* of the frontal lobe controls voluntary movement on the contralateral, or opposite, side of the body. Control areas are arranged topographically so that areas controlling the face are nearest the lateral (Sylvian) fissure, while areas controlling the hip are near the longitudinal fissure. Areas for leg and foot motion are found deep along the inside walls of the longitudinal fissure.

4 Each *parietal lobe* receives sensations from the contralateral side of the body. The parietal lobe of the dominant hemisphere plays a role in calculation, writing, and reading words.

5 The *occipital lobes* are responsible for vision and the ability to recognize objects that are seen.

6 The *temporal lobes* are especially important for the sense of hearing. They also play a role in learning, memory, and emotion. Injury to either temporal lobe can cause aggressive or psychotic behavior or the "hearing" of imaginary sounds. Injury to the temporal lobe of the dominant side can cause failure to understand spoken words.

7 The *cerebellum* maintains the body's sense of balance by combining information from the inner ear (balance receptors) with sight and position sense. The cerebellum also coordinates voluntary body movements.

8 The *spinal cord* meets the brain at the foramen magnum opening of the skull. The spinal cord carries sensations (touch, pain, pressure, temperature sense) from the body to the brain and carries commands for muscle movement from the brain to body muscles.

9 The *medulla* channels information between the cerebral hemispheres and the spinal cord and also controls circulation, heartbeat, and breathing.

Depths and Core

1 A cut into the cerebral hemispheres shows their outermost layer, the *cerebral cortex*, which is made of gray matter. *Gray matter* gets its color from the tightly packed bodies of brain cells (neurons) that live there.

2 White matter lies below the gray matter. *White matter* is made of nerve fibers that form connections between different areas of the cortex. It gets its color from the whitish, fatty covering that surrounds the nerve fibers. White matter also connects the cortex with lower areas of the brain and with the spinal cord.

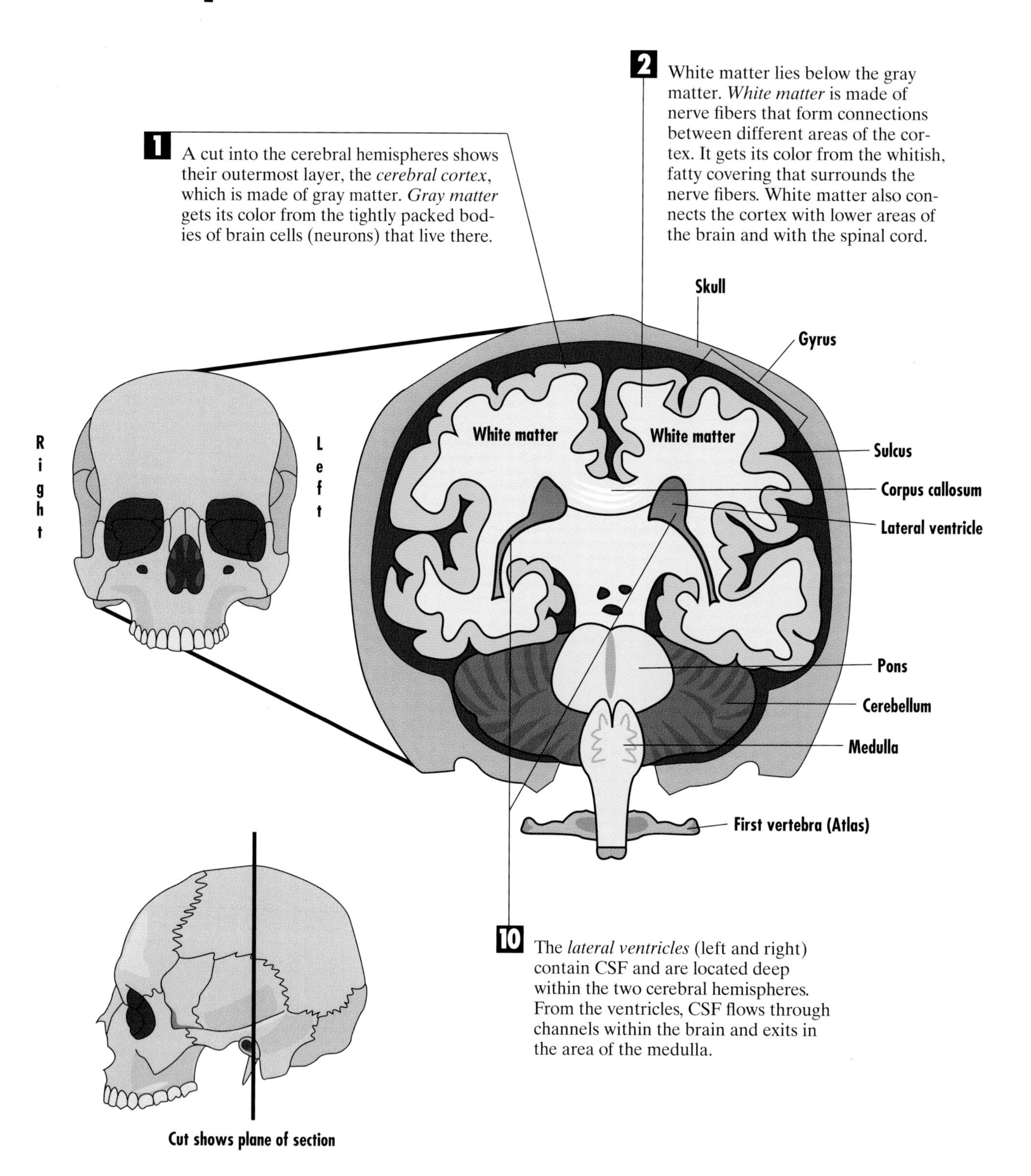

10 The *lateral ventricles* (left and right) contain CSF and are located deep within the two cerebral hemispheres. From the ventricles, CSF flows through channels within the brain and exits in the area of the medulla.

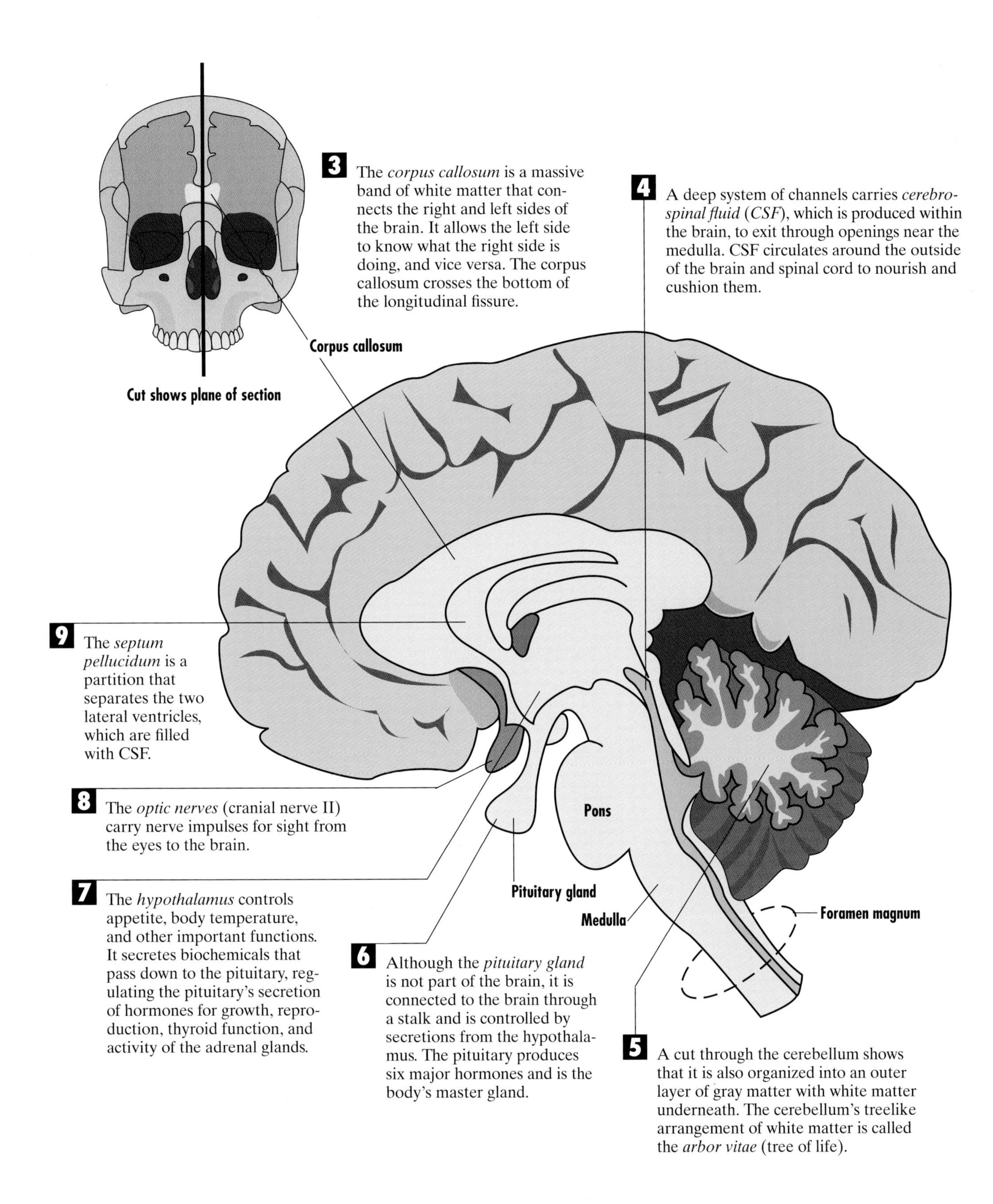
Cut shows plane of section
Corpus callosum
3 The *corpus callosum* is a massive band of white matter that connects the right and left sides of the brain. It allows the left side to know what the right side is doing, and vice versa. The corpus callosum crosses the bottom of the longitudinal fissure.
4 A deep system of channels carries *cerebrospinal fluid* (*CSF*), which is produced within the brain, to exit through openings near the medulla. CSF circulates around the outside of the brain and spinal cord to nourish and cushion them.
9 The *septum pellucidum* is a partition that separates the two lateral ventricles, which are filled with CSF.
8 The *optic nerves* (cranial nerve II) carry nerve impulses for sight from the eyes to the brain.
Pons
Pituitary gland
Medulla
Foramen magnum
7 The *hypothalamus* controls appetite, body temperature, and other important functions. It secretes biochemicals that pass down to the pituitary, regulating the pituitary's secretion of hormones for growth, reproduction, thyroid function, and activity of the adrenal glands.
6 Although the *pituitary gland* is not part of the brain, it is connected to the brain through a stalk and is controlled by secretions from the hypothalamus. The pituitary produces six major hormones and is the body's master gland.
5 A cut through the cerebellum shows that it is also organized into an outer layer of gray matter with white matter underneath. The cerebellum's treelike arrangement of white matter is called the *arbor vitae* (tree of life).

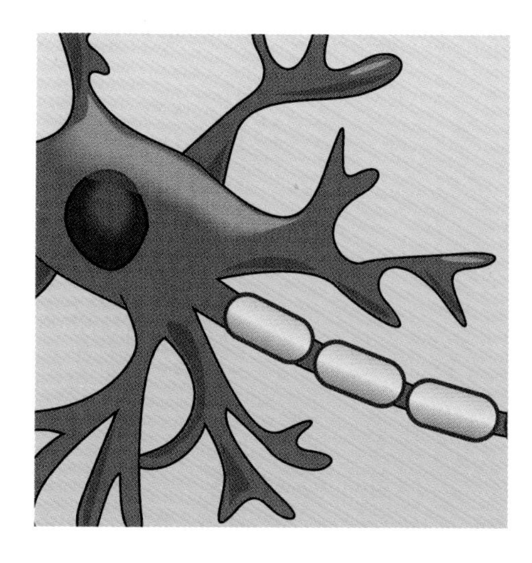

Neuroglia and Neurons

Neural Populations

WHILE EXPLORING THE surface of the brain, you probably wondered why anatomically similar areas of gray matter are functionally different. To explain this, we must meet the local populations.

There are two different types of neural beings, the neuroglia (or glia) and the neurons. *Neuroglia* (about 150 billion of them) have important sustaining roles, but it is the *neurons* (10–15 billion of them) whose actions underlie the brain's higher functions.

Neurons live in the expansive gray matter of the cerebral cortex and in scattered islands of grey matter called nuclei. Neurons have a central cell body that receives input stimulation from branched neuron fibers called dendrites. When a neuron becomes excited by the input it receives, it fires a nerve impulse down its single long output fiber, the axon.

At the axon's endpoint (axon terminal), special biochemical messengers (neurotransmitters) are released. Neurotransmitters can be the input stimulation that excites a neighboring neuron, ultimately generating another nerve impulse in this neighbor. The place where nerve impulses are communicated between consecutive neurons is called a synapse.

Neurons can span great distances with their axons and stimulate (or sometimes inhibit) other neurons far away. It is the axons of neurons that make up the white matter's subterranean communication system. Myelin, fatty insulation around the axons, gives white matter its whiteness.

About 300 million axons make up the *corpus callosum*, the white-matter bridge between the right and left sides of the brain. Smaller bundles of white matter form tracts. Tracts link different parts of the same cerebral hemisphere or link part of the cortex with lower brain areas.

Once the axons reach their destination and discharge their neurotransmitters, nearby neurons receive the biochemical message on areas of their dendrites called receptors. The neurotransmitter capabilities and receptor capabilities of neurons vary from place to place in the brain. So, if we see neurotransmitters as neural words, then neurons speak different languages.

Like the difference between New York City's Wall Street and Broadway, the difference between functional areas of the brain is not so much a matter of geography as it is one of population. It's a reflection of who works there, their interests and goals, their ability to network, their jargon—and the audience they must reach.

Neurons: The Brain's Star Players

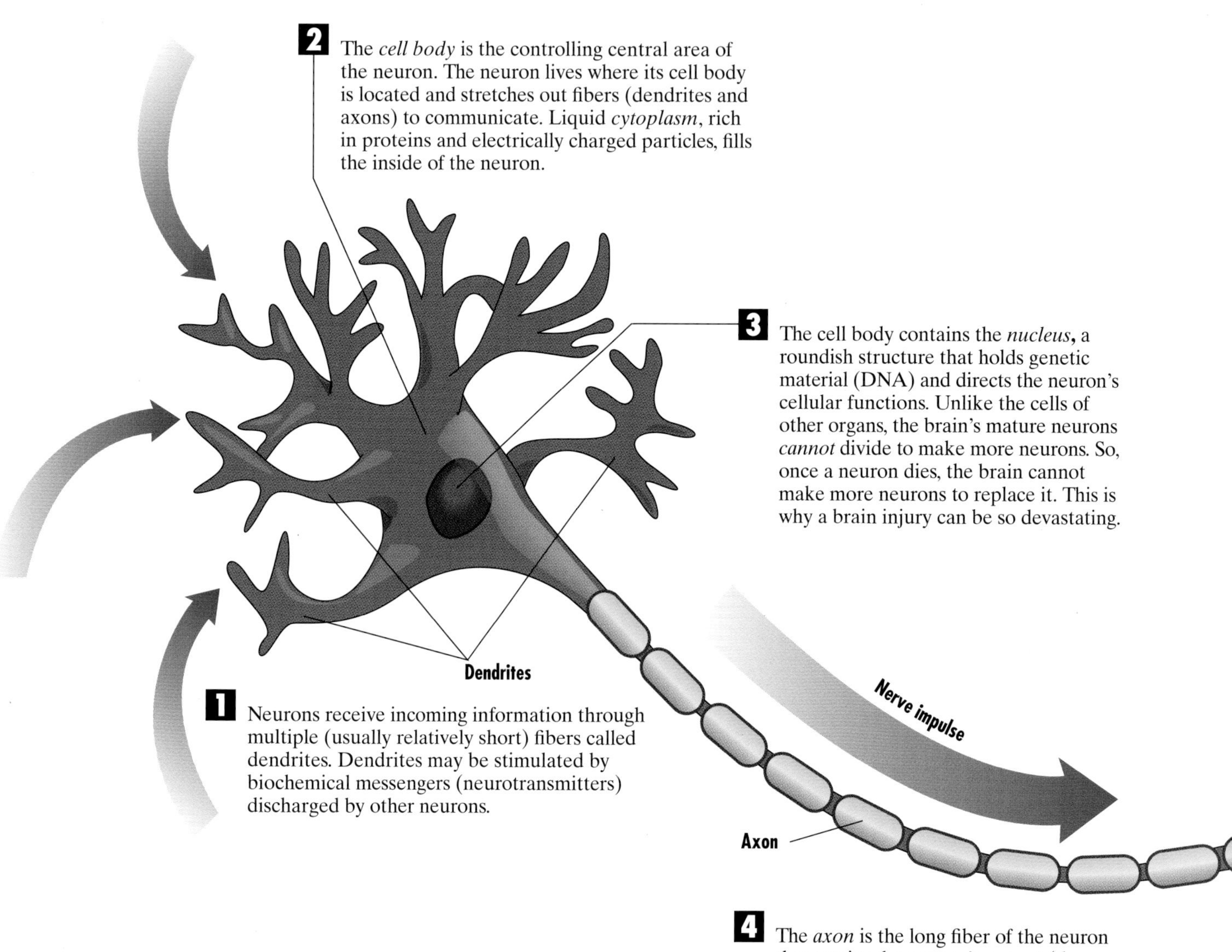

2 The *cell body* is the controlling central area of the neuron. The neuron lives where its cell body is located and stretches out fibers (dendrites and axons) to communicate. Liquid *cytoplasm*, rich in proteins and electrically charged particles, fills the inside of the neuron.

3 The cell body contains the *nucleus*, a roundish structure that holds genetic material (DNA) and directs the neuron's cellular functions. Unlike the cells of other organs, the brain's mature neurons *cannot* divide to make more neurons. So, once a neuron dies, the brain cannot make more neurons to replace it. This is why a brain injury can be so devastating.

1 Neurons receive incoming information through multiple (usually relatively short) fibers called dendrites. Dendrites may be stimulated by biochemical messengers (neurotransmitters) discharged by other neurons.

4 The *axon* is the long fiber of the neuron that carries the neuron's output (the nerve impulse) away from the cell body. Axons can be very long, and those that carry impulses outside the brain can measure more than 1 meter. The axon is covered by a fatty insulation called myelin. Fatty myelin accounts for the white color of the brain's white matter, which is made of many axon fibers lying close together below the brain's gray cortex.

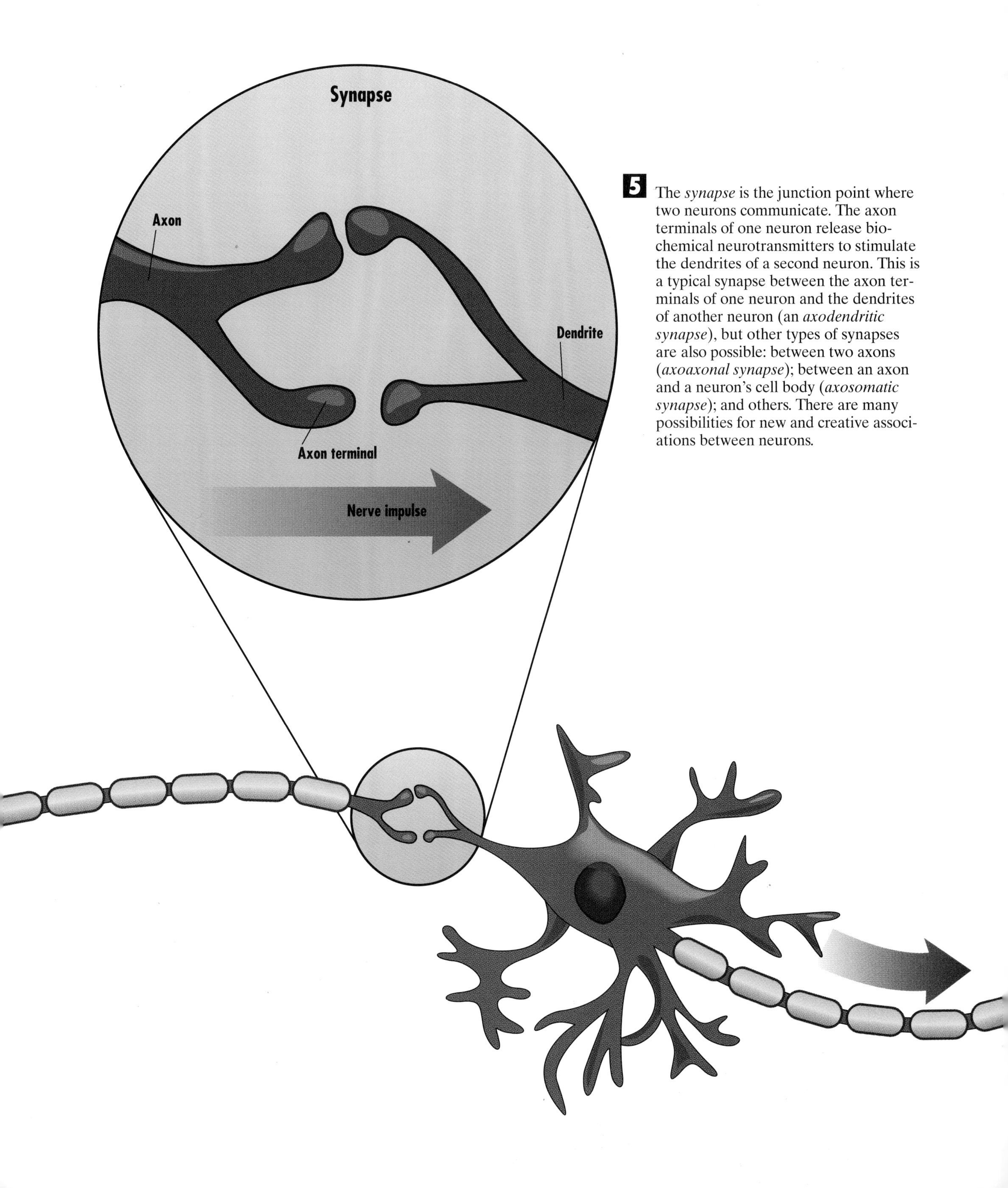

5 The *synapse* is the junction point where two neurons communicate. The axon terminals of one neuron release biochemical neurotransmitters to stimulate the dendrites of a second neuron. This is a typical synapse between the axon terminals of one neuron and the dendrites of another neuron (an *axodendritic synapse*), but other types of synapses are also possible: between two axons (*axoaxonal synapse*); between an axon and a neuron's cell body (*axosomatic synapse*); and others. There are many possibilities for new and creative associations between neurons.

How Nerves Communicate: Nerve Impulse and Synapse

The firing of a nerve impulse begins with a stimulus at the neuron's dendrites. The stimulus is usually a biochemical (a neurotransmitter from another neuron's axon).

1 Neurons live an all-or-nothing lifestyle. They never discharge less than a whole, full nerve impulse. When a stimulus is strong enough to reach a neuron's particular threshold of excitation, the neuron discharges a whole, full nerve impulse. If a stimulus isn't strong enough to reach the threshold, then no nerve impulse is generated at all. Communications between neurons are simple—either On or Off, Yes or No. Neurons don't understand Maybe.

2 The nerve impulse is really an electric phenomenon. It passes down the length of the axon as an abrupt electrical depolarization of the axon's surface membrane. Before the nerve impulse comes, the inside of the axon carries a negative electric charge with respect to the outside. As the nerve impulse arrives, channels open up in the axon's surface membrane and allow a deluge of positively charged ions to flow inside.

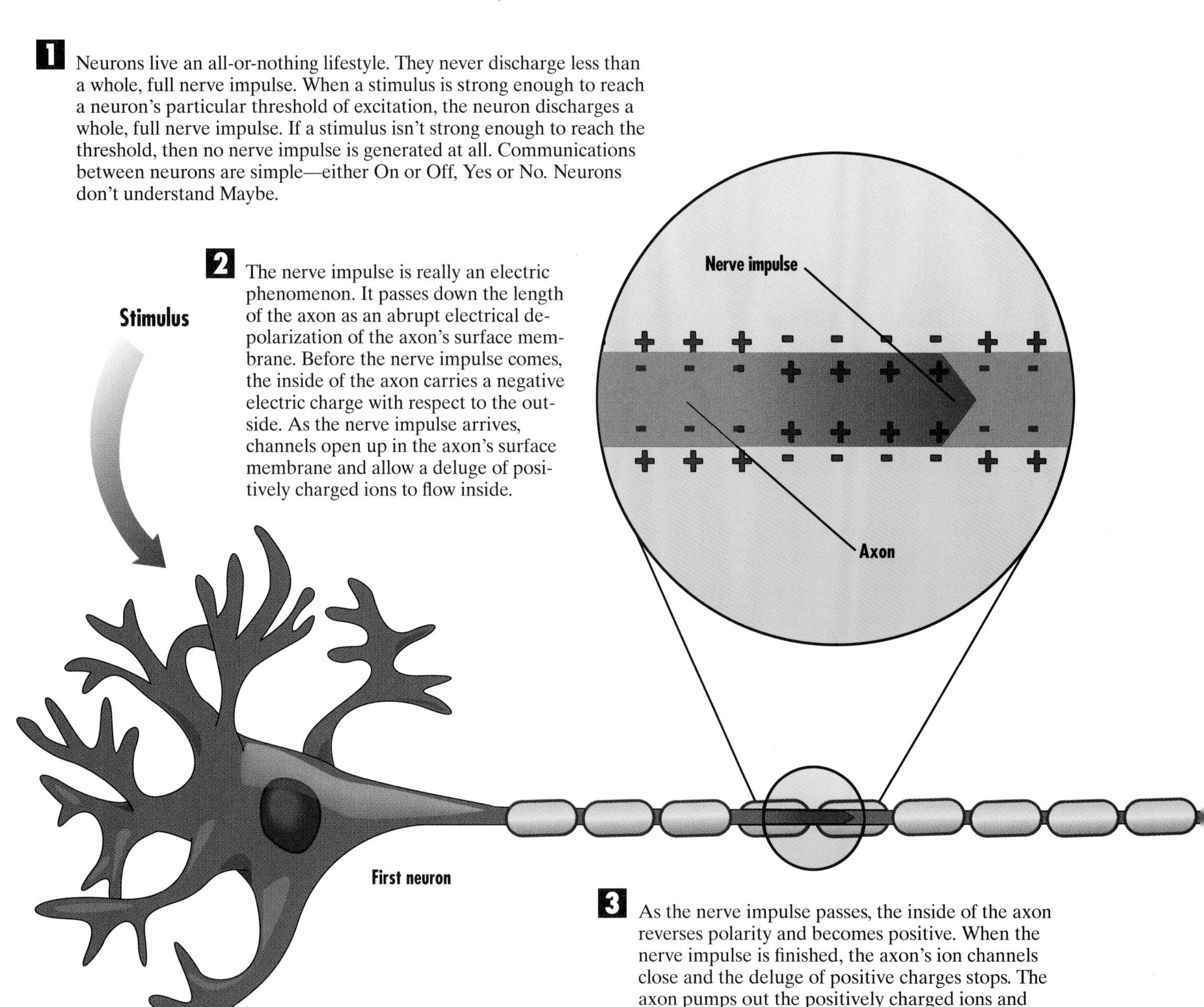

3 As the nerve impulse passes, the inside of the axon reverses polarity and becomes positive. When the nerve impulse is finished, the axon's ion channels close and the deluge of positive charges stops. The axon pumps out the positively charged ions and returns itself to its negative resting state.

4 The axon terminal contains small round packages (*vesicles*) of neurotransmitters that are released when a nerve impulse arrives. Here you see only a few vesicles, but in real life the axon terminal may have thousands.

5 When the electric depolarization of the nerve impulse arrives at the axon terminal, special channels in the surface open up. This allows positively charged calcium ions to rush into the axon.

6 After calcium enters, the axon terminals release their packets of neurotransmitters. Neurotransmitter molecules travel across the *synaptic cleft* (space between axon and dendrite) to reach receptors on the dendrites of our second neuron. This journey takes 4 milliseconds or less.

7 Neurotransmitters bind to *receptor sites* on the outside membrane of the dendrite. Receptor sites are very specific, so they fit some neurotransmitters but not others.

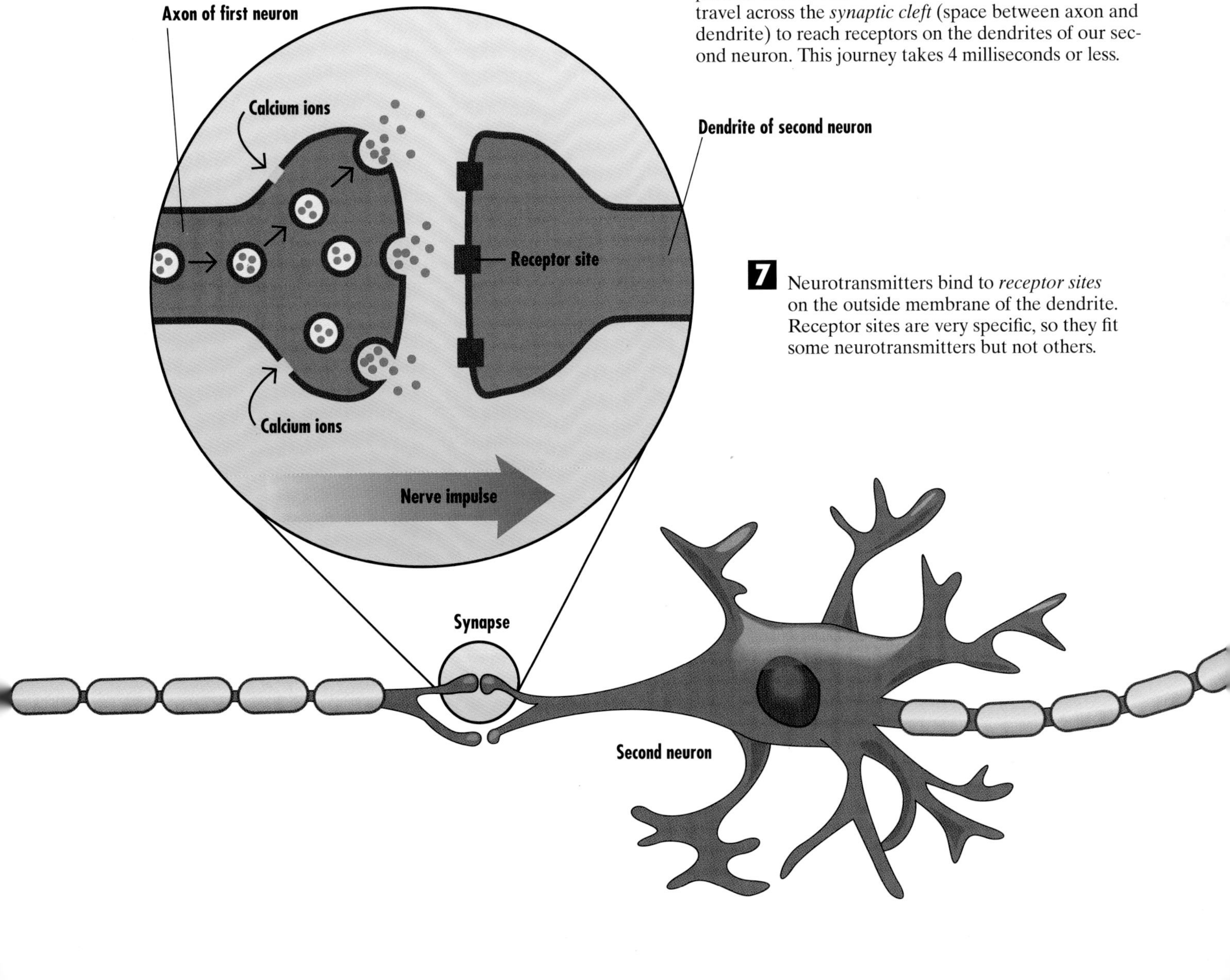

Neuron Relationships: Tracts and Neurotransmitters

1 Billions of axon fibers in the white matter form the communication cables that link one part of the brain to another. Fibers with the same origin and destination travel in bundles called tracts. Here we see just a few of the many association tracts of the brain. These link one part of the cortex's gray matter to another within the same hemisphere, left or right. In earlier illustrations we saw the corpus callosum, a major communications link between the hemispheres.

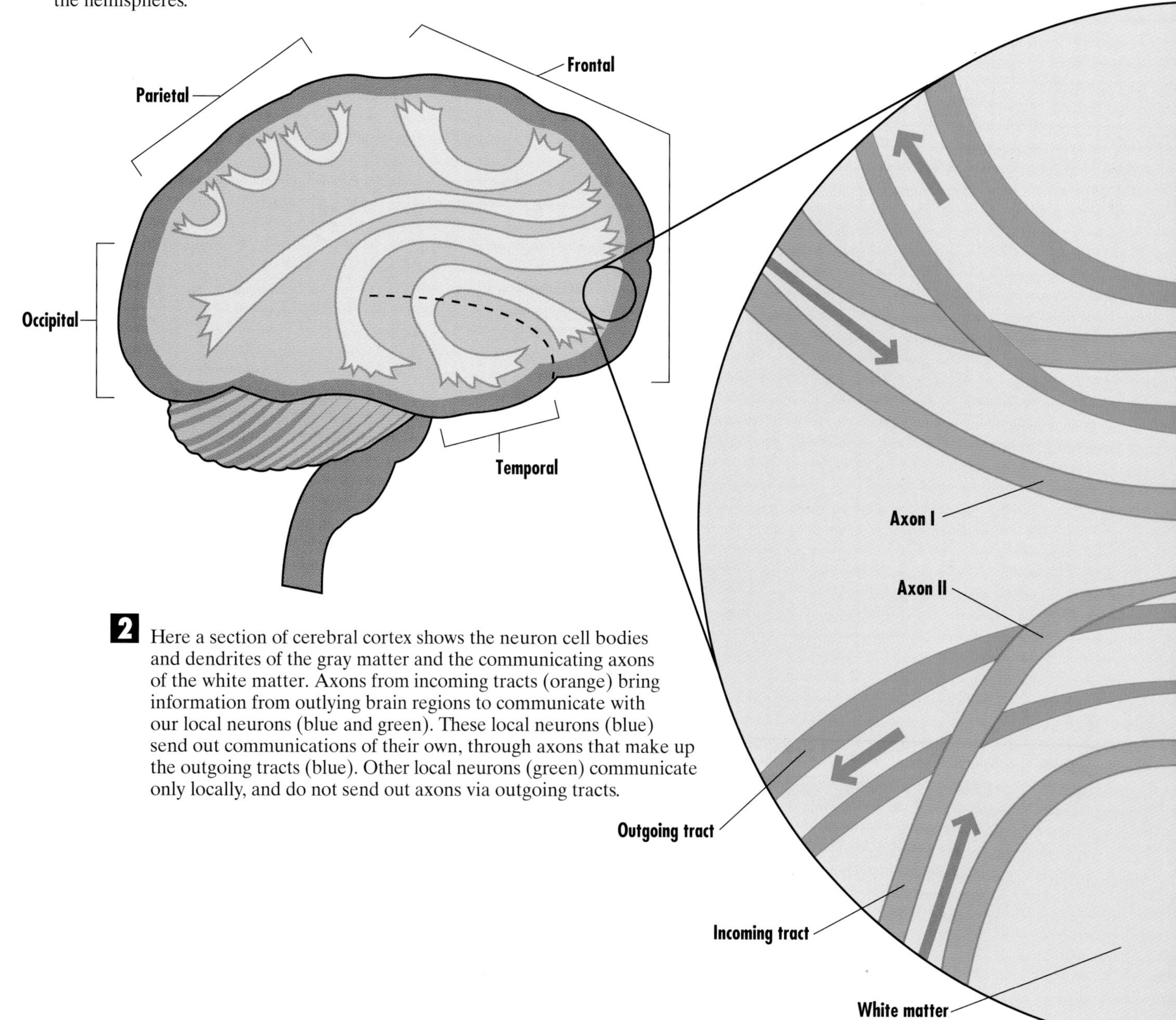

2 Here a section of cerebral cortex shows the neuron cell bodies and dendrites of the gray matter and the communicating axons of the white matter. Axons from incoming tracts (orange) bring information from outlying brain regions to communicate with our local neurons (blue and green). These local neurons (blue) send out communications of their own, through axons that make up the outgoing tracts (blue). Other local neurons (green) communicate only locally, and do not send out axons via outgoing tracts.

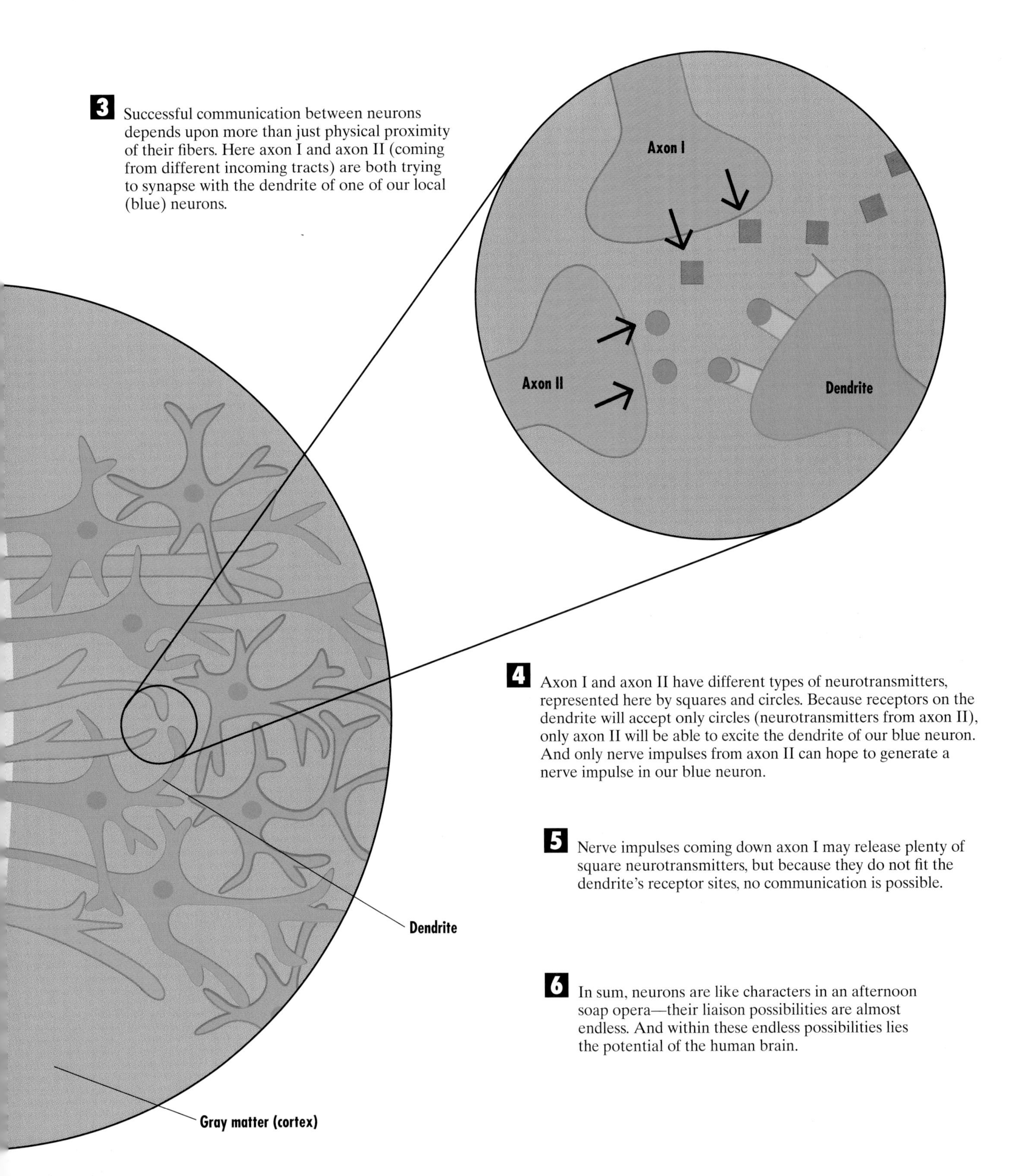

3 Successful communication between neurons depends upon more than just physical proximity of their fibers. Here axon I and axon II (coming from different incoming tracts) are both trying to synapse with the dendrite of one of our local (blue) neurons.

4 Axon I and axon II have different types of neurotransmitters, represented here by squares and circles. Because receptors on the dendrite will accept only circles (neurotransmitters from axon II), only axon II will be able to excite the dendrite of our blue neuron. And only nerve impulses from axon II can hope to generate a nerve impulse in our blue neuron.

5 Nerve impulses coming down axon I may release plenty of square neurotransmitters, but because they do not fit the dendrite's receptor sites, no communication is possible.

6 In sum, neurons are like characters in an afternoon soap opera—their liaison possibilities are almost endless. And within these endless possibilities lies the potential of the human brain.

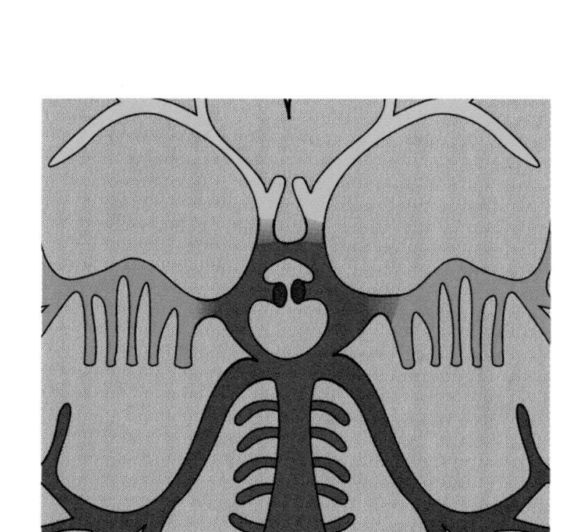

Oxygen and Blood Supply Lines

Energy for the Neural World

BECAUSE THE NEURAL population lives a very active life, the brain requires a constant and steady supply of both nutritional energy (food) and oxygen. Neither one of these commodities is produced or effectively stored in the brain, so each must be imported on a planetary scale. It is the brain's circulation that provides the major supply lines for all its life-sustaining imports.

Since neurons may die after 5 minutes without oxygen, the brain's survival depends upon efficient oxygen supply lines from the lungs. Likewise, since the brain's primary food source is glucose (a simple sugar), the brain must constantly draw its supply from the body's biggest producer of blood sugar, the liver. To assure an uninterrupted supply of blood from both the lungs and liver, the brain relies on the heart and on an efficient—and structurally intriguing—circulation pattern.

All blood comes to the brain through the neck, mainly through the carotid arteries (traveling unprotected in the front of the neck), and the vertebral arteries (protected by bony tunnels in the spine). At the bottom of the brain, major incoming blood vessels feed the brain's Circle of Willis.

The *Circle of Willis* is a remarkable construction. It links the brain's major arteries like highways in a traffic circle and effectively channels incoming blood along diverging routes to the front, middle, and back of the brain. In the event of a severe blockage within the circle, there exists an anatomic potential for rerouting and flow compensation.

Anything imported into the brain through the bloodstream goes through the brain's equivalent of customs, the *blood-brain barrier*. This barrier has two components—the molecularly tight walls of the brain's smallest blood vessels, and the astrocytes (a type of neuroglia). These two components allow only select molecules (like glucose, the energy source) to pass into the brain.

Also from the circulatory system comes the brain's protective atmosphere, the *cerebrospinal fluid* (CSF). CSF is produced in cavernlike ventricles lying deep inside the brain. It is filtered from the bloodstream in highly vascular areas, the choroid plexuses. CSF travels through the brain's subterranean caverns and ultimately springs up to the brain's surface near the medulla. From there it percolates through the subarachnoid space (between the meninges) and surrounds the brain.

CSF forms the brain's watery surface environment. Like a car's protective air bag, the CSF provides a shock-absorbing cushion around the brain, shielding it from impact against the inside of the skull.

Supply Lines: Circulation and the Blood-Brain Barrier

5 One vertebral artery runs on each side of the spine to bring blood to the brain. The right and left vertebral arteries join at the bottom of the brain to form the basilar artery, which contributes incoming blood to the Circle of Willis.

Internal carotid artery

4 The carotid arteries (pulsing at each side of the front of the neck) send large branches (the right and left internal carotid arteries) into the brain. The internal carotid arteries bring incoming blood to the Circle of Willis.

3 The heart pumps blood from the lungs and liver to the brain. If the heart stops (cardiac arrest), unconsciousness usually results within 10 seconds.

2 The liver maintains normal levels of glucose, the brain's main fuel. If the glucose level drops, the liver can manufacture more, even by breaking down muscle protein.

1 The lungs are responsible for the brain's oxygen supply. A decreased oxygen level can cause inattention, impaired judgement, and coordination problems. Complete lack of oxygen can kill the brain's neurons within 5 minutes.

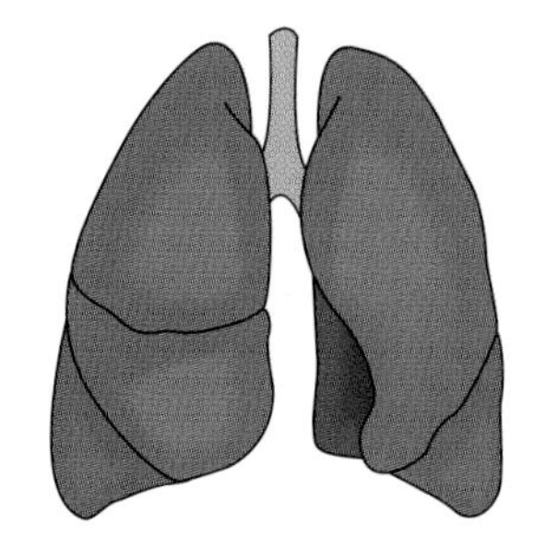

6 The Circle of Willis links many important arteries within the brain. There are equivalent anterior, middle, and posterior cerebral arteries for both the left and right hemispheres.

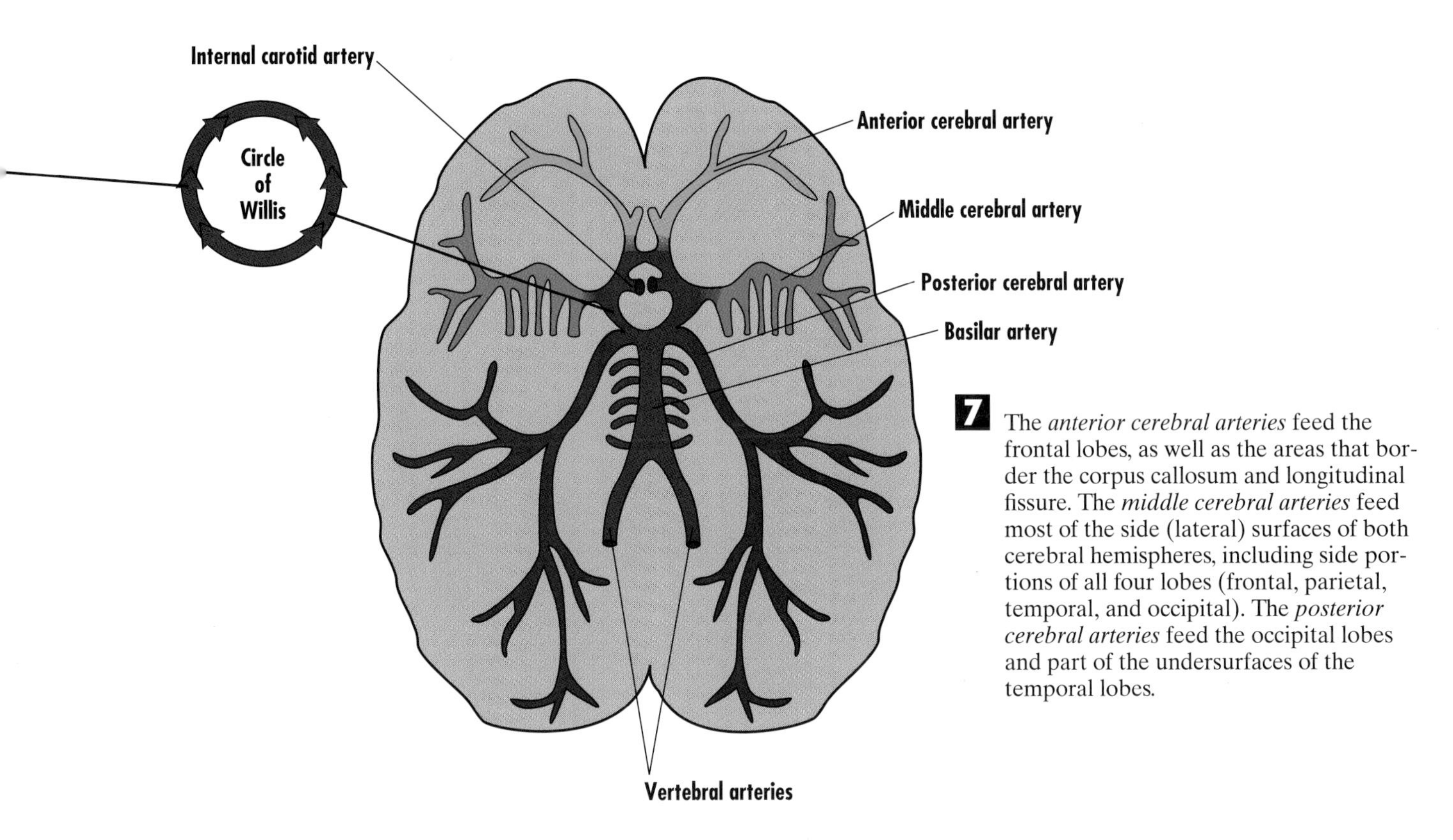

7 The *anterior cerebral arteries* feed the frontal lobes, as well as the areas that border the corpus callosum and longitudinal fissure. The *middle cerebral arteries* feed most of the side (lateral) surfaces of both cerebral hemispheres, including side portions of all four lobes (frontal, parietal, temporal, and occipital). The *posterior cerebral arteries* feed the occipital lobes and part of the undersurfaces of the temporal lobes.

8 The blood-brain barrier is the brain's protective customs service. It is not a physical wall, but a series of screening measures. It allows only selected chemicals to pass from the bloodstream into the brain.

9 The first part of the blood-brain barrier is formed by cells that line the walls of the brain's smallest blood vessels. The junctions between these cells are very tight and act to exclude many larger molecules.

10 *Astrocytes* (one type of neuroglia) use their "feet" to attach themselves to the outside of neighboring blood vessels. Astrocytes appear to further screen chemicals that have already passed through the vessel walls.

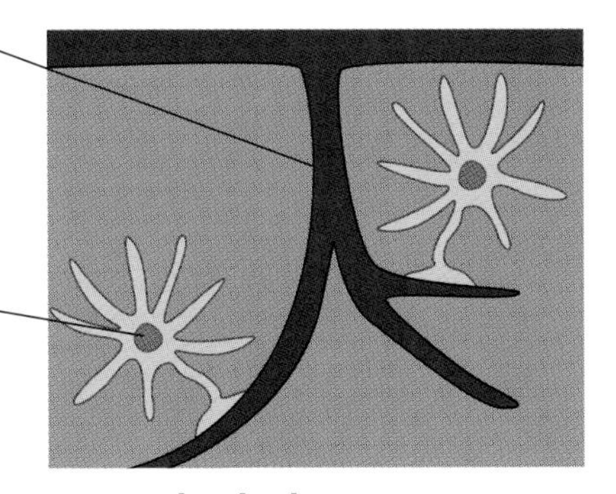

The Blood-Brain Barrier

From the Caverns Comes Protection: The Cerebral Spinal Fluid

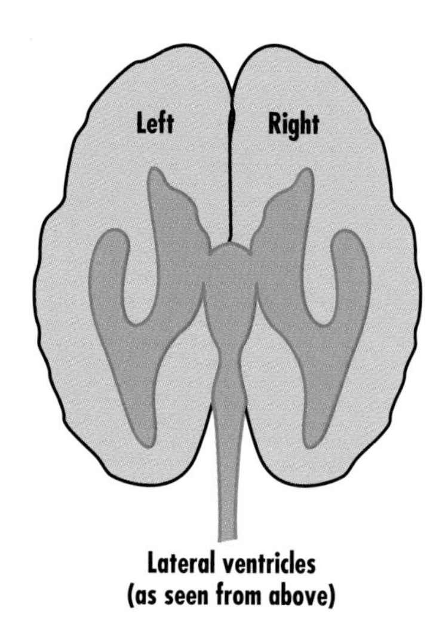

Lateral ventricles
(as seen from above)

1 There is a total of 125–150 milliliters of cerebrospinal fluid (CSF) surrounding the brain and spinal cord and filling the brain's internal system of ventricles. CSF cushions the brain and spinal cord from impact against the inside of the bony skull and spinal canal.

2 The two lateral ventricles, one in each cerebral hemisphere, are cavernous spaces filled with CSF. Within each lateral ventricle, the *choroid plexus* produces clear CSF from red blood flowing through a rich supply of blood vessels. Up to 700 milliliters of CSF is produced every day. This circulates around the brain and spinal cord and then is reabsorbed into the circulation. From the lateral ventricles, CSF flows to the centrally located third ventricle.

3 The third ventricle also has a choroid plexus (red) on its roof, where more CSF is produced. From the third ventricle, CSF flows through the tubular cerebral aqueduct (aqueduct of Sylvius) to the fourth ventricle.

4 The *foramina of Luschka* (one on each side, right and left) are small portals where CSF passes to the brain's surface.

5 The *foramen of Magendie*, on the roof of the fourth ventricle, is another exit for CSF traveling to the brain's surface. On the surface of the brain the CSF percolates through the subarachnoid space between the layers of meninges.

6 The appearance and chemical composition of CSF is important in diagnosing certain types of brain illness. CSF from the spinal area can be used because the same CSF that circulates around the surface of the brain also surrounds the spinal cord. In the area of the lower spine it is relatively safe to remove some CSF with a hollow needle without damaging the spinal cord. This sterile diagnostic procedure is called a lumbar puncture (LP).

8 A close-up view of an arachnoid villus also allows us to see the meninges. The meninges have three layers: the pia mater, the arachnoid, and the dura mater. The *pia mater* contains many tiny blood vessels and adheres closely to the surface of the brain and spinal cord. The *arachnoid*, the middle layer of the meninges, has a fine texture like a spider's web. CSF flows between the arachnoid and the pia mater in the subarachnoid space. The arachnoid villi are projections of the arachnoid layer of the meninges. The *dura mater* is the tough outermost layer of the meninges.

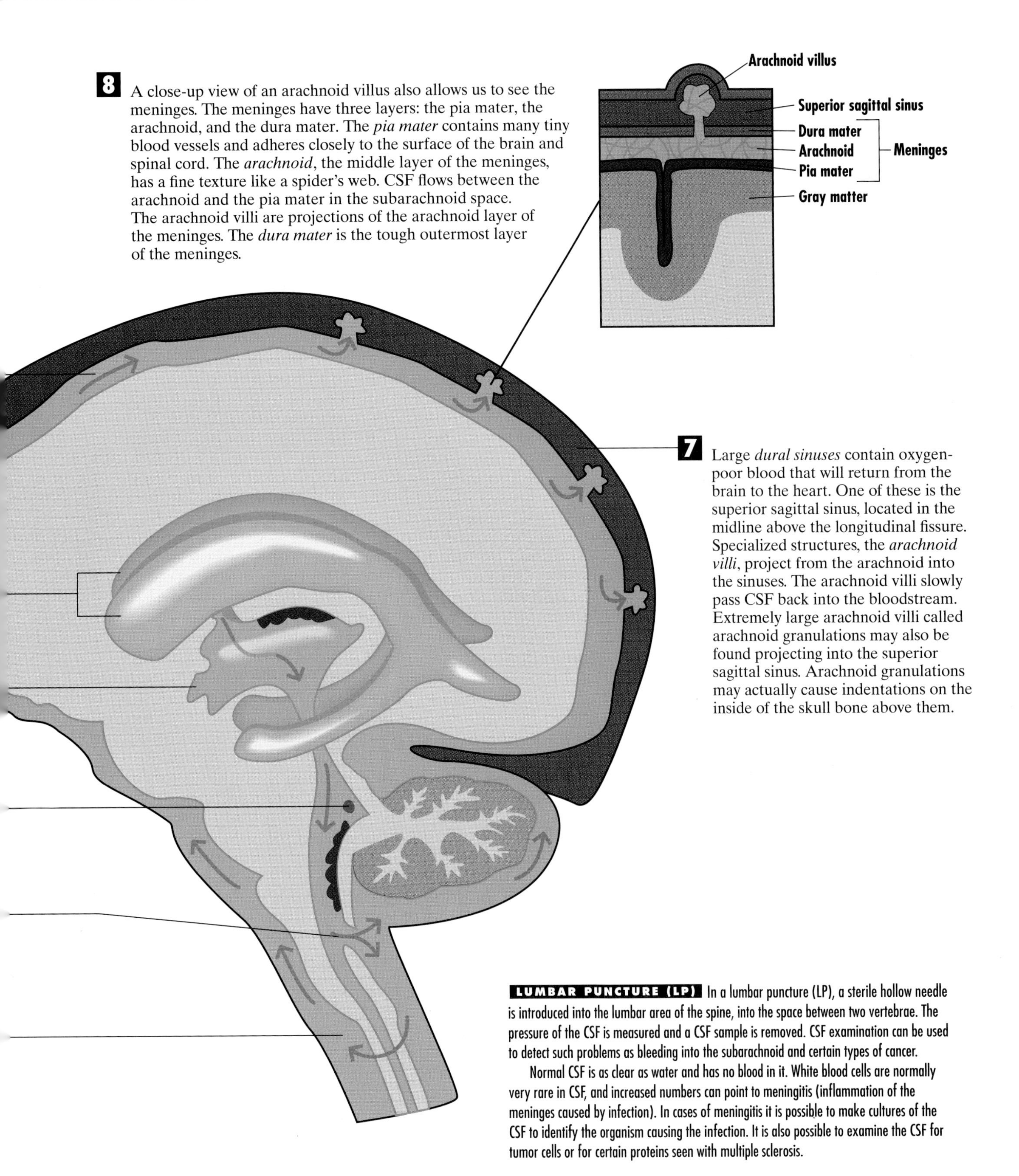

7 Large *dural sinuses* contain oxygen-poor blood that will return from the brain to the heart. One of these is the superior sagittal sinus, located in the midline above the longitudinal fissure. Specialized structures, the *arachnoid villi*, project from the arachnoid into the sinuses. The arachnoid villi slowly pass CSF back into the bloodstream. Extremely large arachnoid villi called arachnoid granulations may also be found projecting into the superior sagittal sinus. Arachnoid granulations may actually cause indentations on the inside of the skull bone above them.

LUMBAR PUNCTURE (LP) In a lumbar puncture (LP), a sterile hollow needle is introduced into the lumbar area of the spine, into the space between two vertebrae. The pressure of the CSF is measured and a CSF sample is removed. CSF examination can be used to detect such problems as bleeding into the subarachnoid and certain types of cancer.

Normal CSF is as clear as water and has no blood in it. White blood cells are normally very rare in CSF, and increased numbers can point to meningitis (inflammation of the meninges caused by infection). In cases of meningitis it is possible to make cultures of the CSF to identify the organism causing the infection. It is also possible to examine the CSF for tumor cells or for certain proteins seen with multiple sclerosis.

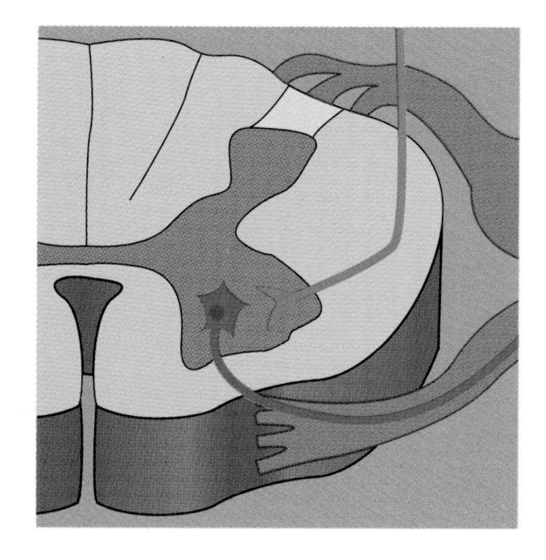

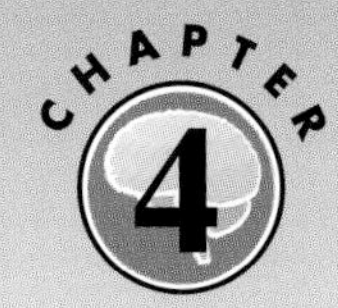

The Spinal Cord
A Neural Media Network

IN ORDER TO survive, the brain must maintain a complex media network for gathering sensory information on which to base its reactions. General sensations for touch, pain, pressure, and temperature are reported to the brain via the spinal cord, the main conduit of information to and from the brain. The special senses—sight, hearing, smell, taste—as well as facial sensations are reported via cranial nerves (see Chapter 7).

The spinal cord is continuous with the brain at the foramen magnum, but its white matter and gray matter locations are reversed (gray inside, white outside). As in the brain, the spinal cord's white matter is formed by tracts of neuron fibers covered with fatty myelin. These tracts pass up and down the spinal cord. They carry sensory information to the brain, and they bring the brain's motor responses (directions for movement) down to the muscles.

Sensory information from the skin, joints, and muscles is gathered by specialized receptors at the ends of sensory neurons. Sensory neuron receptors have distinct structural appearances and report different types of stimuli—pain, pressure, temperature, and various "touch" sensations. Different sensations travel via different white matter tracts to the brain. Receptors fire continuously and simultaneously all over the body, sending a complex barrage of media information to the brain. Some of this information (such as the sensation of wearing comfortable shoes), can be selectively and safely ignored, while some of it (the feeling that a nail has gone through the sole of your shoe) demands response.

In response to sensory information brought via the spinal cord, the brain sends motor responses to the muscles of the body. About 1 million neurons in the precentral gyrus (frontal lobe) send their axons down the spinal cord via descending tracts of white matter fibers. Their goal is to make contact with motor neurons that control the body's muscles, and they may reach out to neurons on more than one level of the cord along their way.

For the sake of simplicity, we will follow the path of only one sensory tract to the brain, and we will travel only one motor tract back. There are really many more tracts in each direction. Also, within the spinal cord itself, there are synapses and interconnecting pathways that vastly increase the number of possible associations. These associations magnify the brain's sensory experience and help it to respond with self-expressive body movements.

How the Spinal Cord Conducts Information

1 The spinal cord is the main conduit for information going to and from the brain. Between the bony vertebrae that protect it, the spinal cord is able to send out spinal nerves for communication with the body. There are 31 pairs of spinal nerves, and each pair arises from a specific region of the spinal cord: *cervical* (from the neck region), *thoracic* (from the rib region), *lumbar* (from the middle part of the back), *sacral* (from the lower back), and *coccygeal* (near the tailbone).

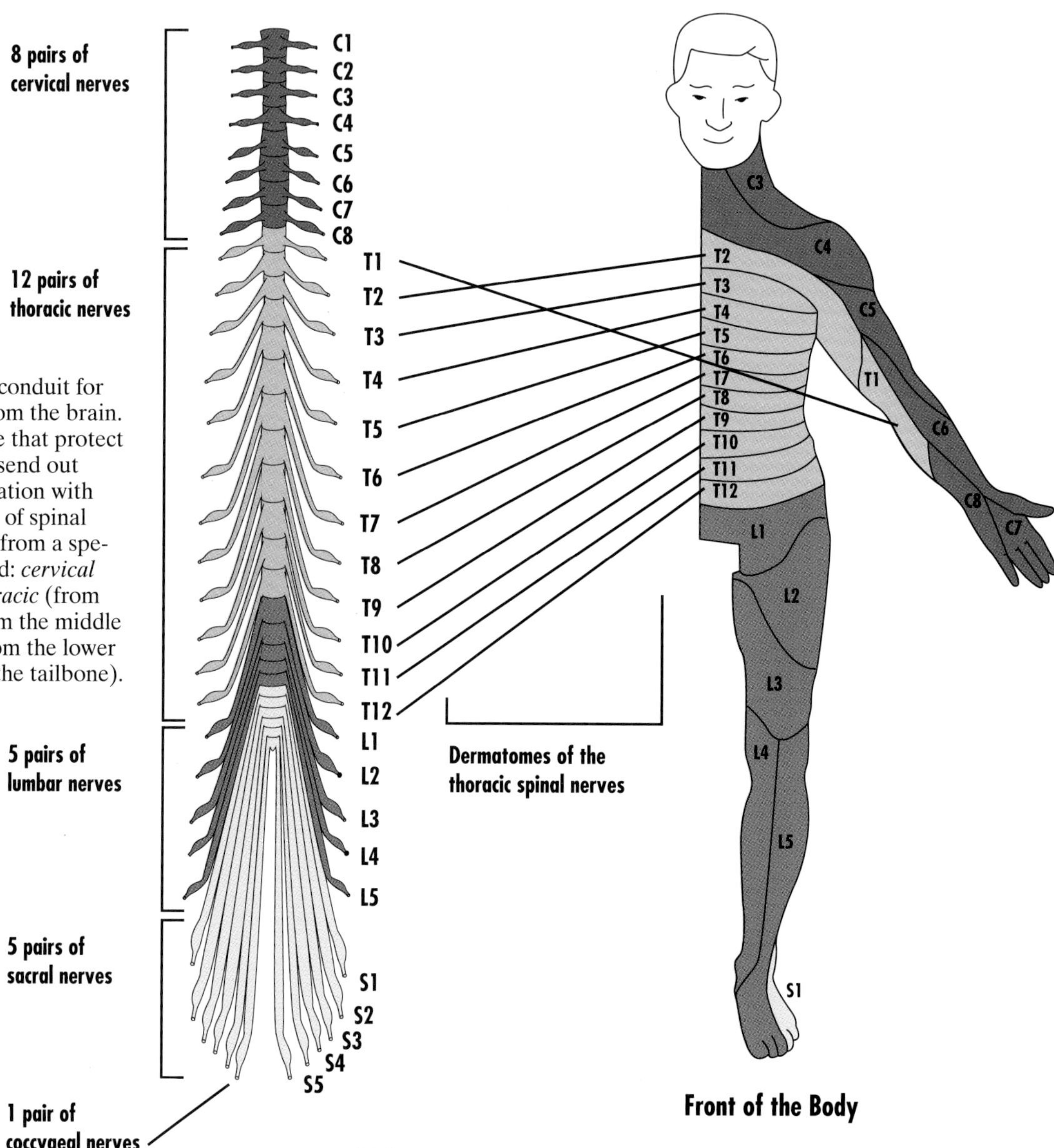

2 Spinal nerves are not distributed to body regions at random. Specific spinal nerves receive sensations from specific areas of the body; these areas are called *dermatomes*. For example, the dermatome area that sends sensations into the tenth thoracic spinal nerve (T10) is located at approximately the level of the navel. Here we see the thoracic spinal nerves correlated with the position of their respective dermatomes on the front of the body. There are dermatomes for the back of the body, as well.

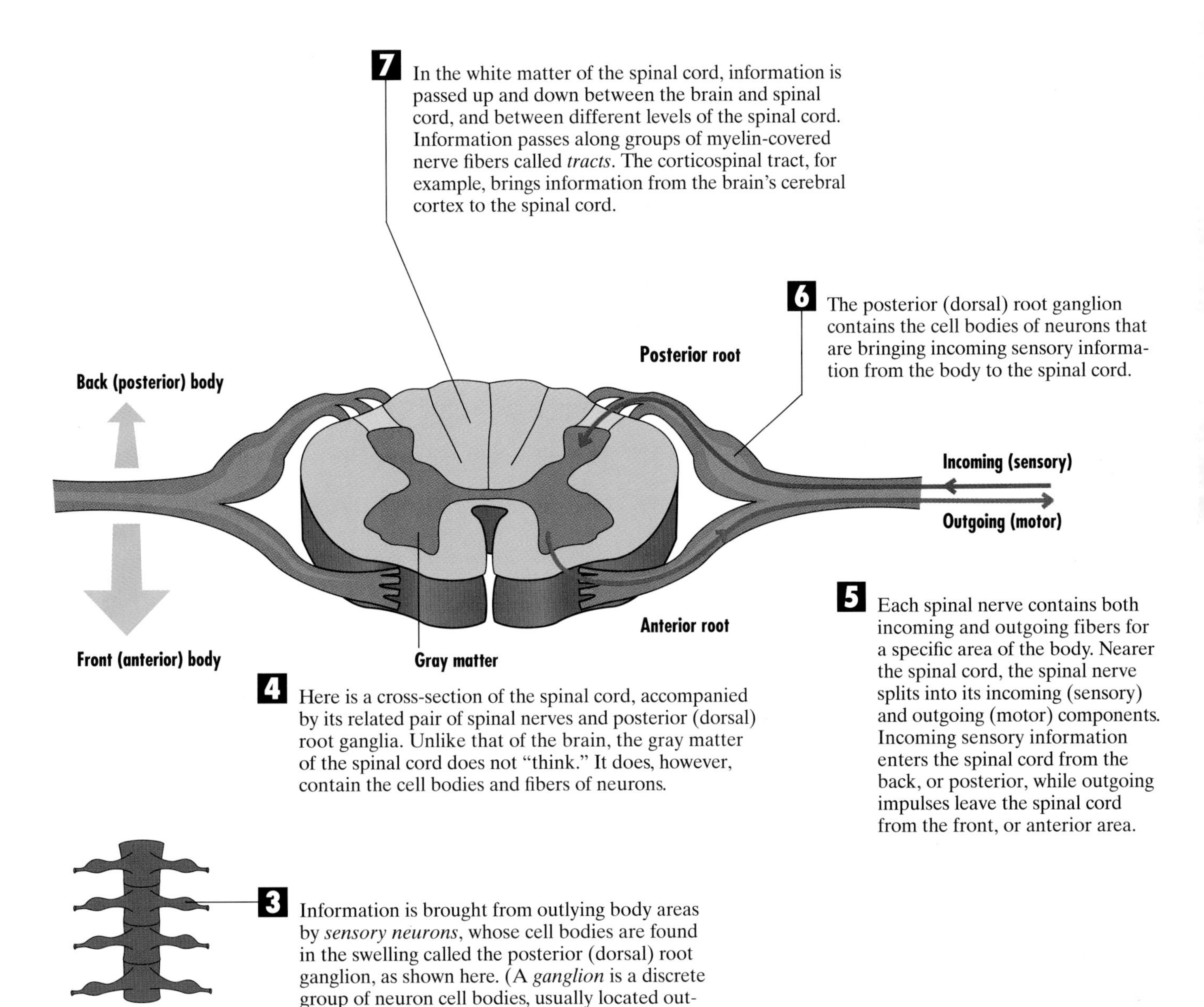

7 In the white matter of the spinal cord, information is passed up and down between the brain and spinal cord, and between different levels of the spinal cord. Information passes along groups of myelin-covered nerve fibers called *tracts*. The corticospinal tract, for example, brings information from the brain's cerebral cortex to the spinal cord.

6 The posterior (dorsal) root ganglion contains the cell bodies of neurons that are bringing incoming sensory information from the body to the spinal cord.

4 Here is a cross-section of the spinal cord, accompanied by its related pair of spinal nerves and posterior (dorsal) root ganglia. Unlike that of the brain, the gray matter of the spinal cord does not "think." It does, however, contain the cell bodies and fibers of neurons.

5 Each spinal nerve contains both incoming and outgoing fibers for a specific area of the body. Nearer the spinal cord, the spinal nerve splits into its incoming (sensory) and outgoing (motor) components. Incoming sensory information enters the spinal cord from the back, or posterior, while outgoing impulses leave the spinal cord from the front, or anterior area.

3 Information is brought from outlying body areas by *sensory neurons*, whose cell bodies are found in the swelling called the posterior (dorsal) root ganglion, as shown here. (A *ganglion* is a discrete group of neuron cell bodies, usually located outside the brain or spinal cord.)

The Sensory Neuron: From Stimulus to Sensation

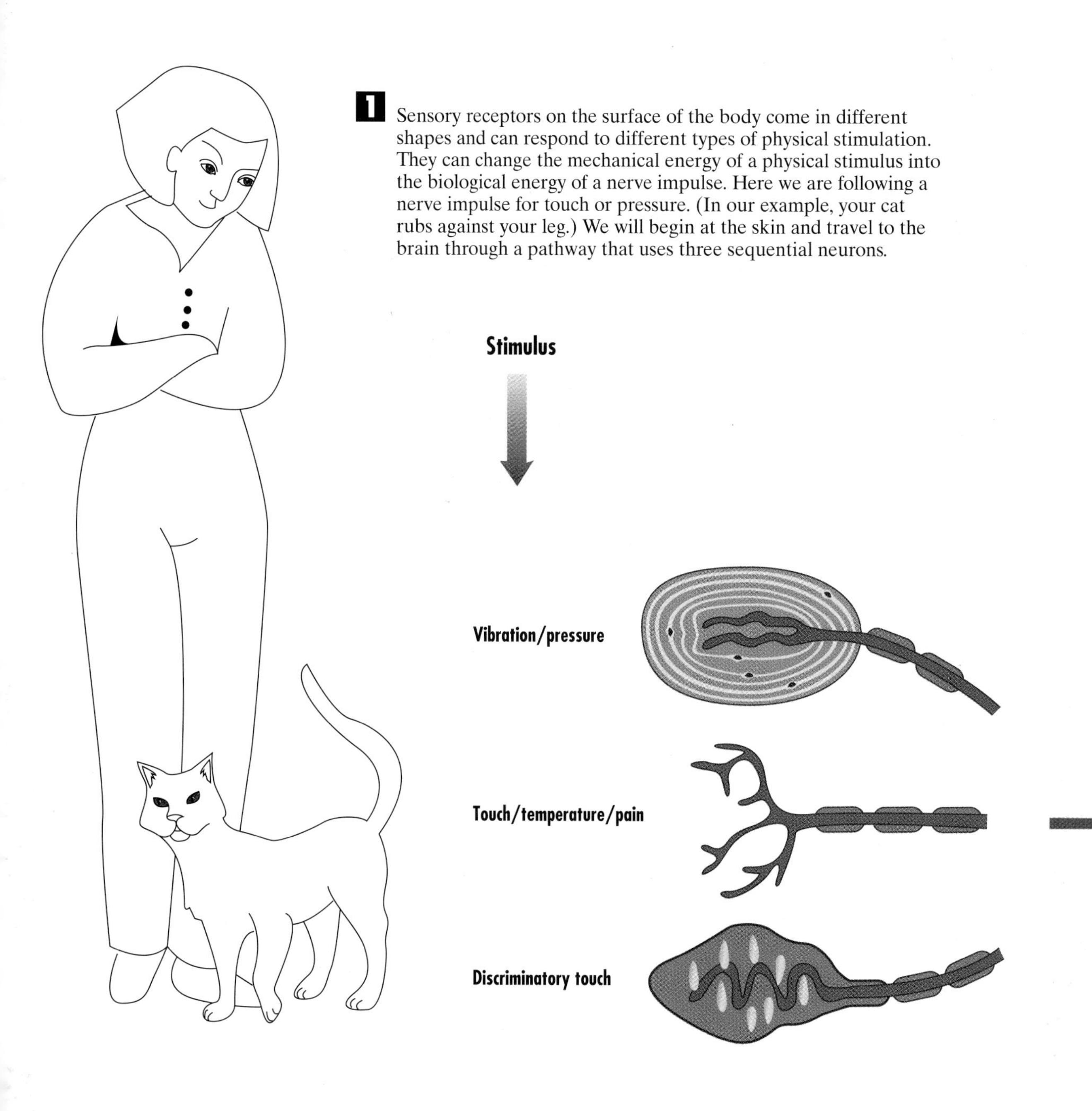

1 Sensory receptors on the surface of the body come in different shapes and can respond to different types of physical stimulation. They can change the mechanical energy of a physical stimulus into the biological energy of a nerve impulse. Here we are following a nerve impulse for touch or pressure. (In our example, your cat rubs against your leg.) We will begin at the skin and travel to the brain through a pathway that uses three sequential neurons.

Postcentral Gyrus The postcentral gyrus is the area of the parietal lobe immediately behind the central sulcus. It is a major reception area for sensations from all parts of the body. In general, the sensations received are contralateral, with the postcentral gyrus of the left parietal lobe receiving sensations from the right side of the body, and vice versa.

5 In the last part of the sensory journey, Neuron III carries the sensory nerve impulse to the cerebral cortex. It ends in the postcentral gyrus of the parietal lobe. Sensation: You feel the touch of fur and the pressure of your cat's body.

Sensation

4 Neuron II carries the nerve impulse to the *thalamus*, a deep area of the brain located near the third ventricle. The thalamus has an important role as a relay station, and it is here that Neuron II synapses with Neuron III (red).

Thalamus (a deep structure)

3 The first synapse along this sensory pathway occurs in the medulla of the brain. Neuron I synapses with Neuron II (pink) and the sensory impulse is passed on. While traveling through the medulla, Neuron II crosses from one side to the other, carrying the nerve impulse with it. This crossing in the medulla causes sensory stimuli from the right side of the body to be received by the left side of the brain, and vice versa.

Medulla

Foramen magnum of skull

Spinal cord

2 Neuron I (blue) receives the nerve impulse from its receptor endings in the skin. The nerve impulse passes to the neuron's cell body, which is located in a posterior (dorsal) root ganglion. The nerve impulse continues along the outgoing fiber of Neuron I, through the white matter of the spinal cord's posterior funiculus and all the way up to the medulla of the brain. Notice that the path from the skin to the medulla was accomplished using only Neuron I, without a synapse. Consequently, sensory neurons like Neuron I need to be very long; some are longer than 2 meters.

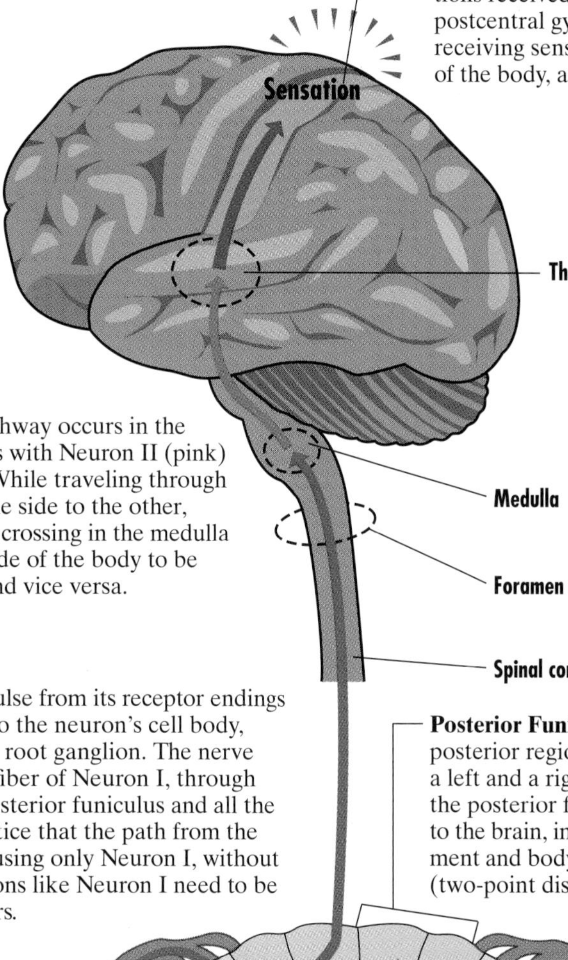

Posterior Funiculus White matter along the posterior region of the spinal cord forms both a left and a right posterior funiculus. Tracts in the posterior funiculi carry several sensations to the brain, including sensation of body movement and body position and discrete touch (two-point discrimination).

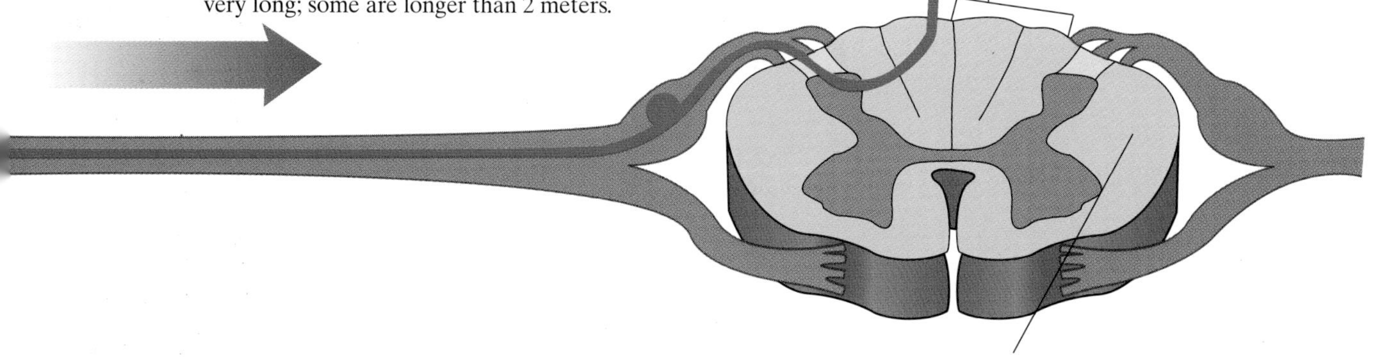

Lateral Funiculus On each side of the spinal cord, white matter forms the right and the left lateral funiculus. Sensory tracts running in the lateral funiculus carry pain and temperature sensations to the brain.

The Motor Neuron: Reaction!

1 Now that you know there is a cat rubbing against your leg, what are you going to do about it? Here we trace the pathway of a neuron bringing the message for voluntary muscle control. We are traveling on the corticospinal tract, from the cerebral cortex to the spinal cord. We start at the precentral gyrus of the frontal lobe and end at the muscle fibers of a voluntary muscle. In the pre-central gyrus the brain "thinks" that it wants to move a muscle (to pet the cat) and a nerve impulse is generated. The reason for any voluntary motion is up to the individual brain—the command for motion may be grossly the same whether we are trying a new dance step or stepping on a cockroach.

Pons

Medulla

2 The nerve impulse (orange) for muscle movement (a motor impulse) travels down to the spinal cord via only one neuron, without making a synapse. Usually (up to 90% of the time), in the area where the brain and spinal cord meet, fibers of the corticospinal tract change sides. Fibers that originated in the right cerebral cortex now cross to the left side of the spinal cord, and vice versa.

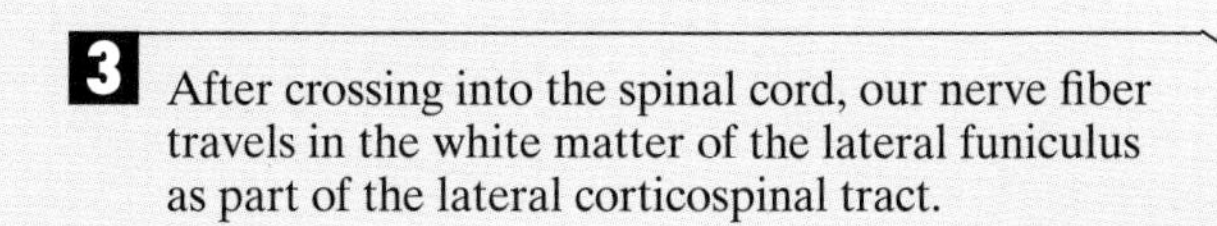

3 After crossing into the spinal cord, our nerve fiber travels in the white matter of the lateral funiculus as part of the lateral corticospinal tract.

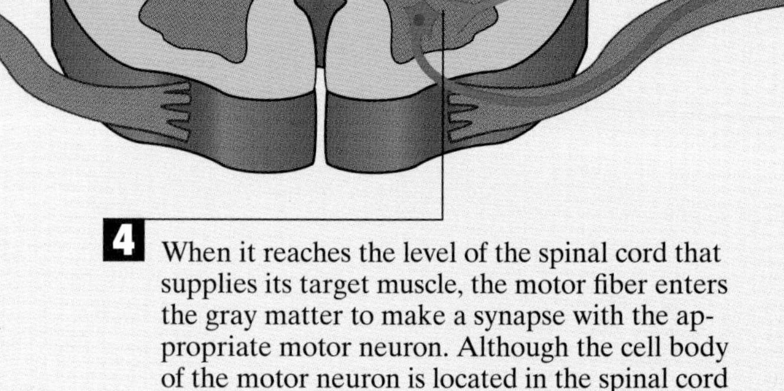

4 When it reaches the level of the spinal cord that supplies its target muscle, the motor fiber enters the gray matter to make a synapse with the appropriate motor neuron. Although the cell body of the motor neuron is located in the spinal cord gray matter, its fibers reach out over considerable distances to contact body muscles.

MOTOR NEURON DISEASE Because a skeletal muscle will waste away if it loses its motor neuron, muscle weakness and wasting can be signs of motor neuron disease. The most common form of progressive motor neuron disease is *amyotrophic lateral sclerosis (ALS)*. ALS affects about 2 out of every 100,000 persons worldwide, and is hereditary in 5%–10% of cases. It begins with insidious muscle weakness and wasting, and it ends in death. There is currently no effective treatment.

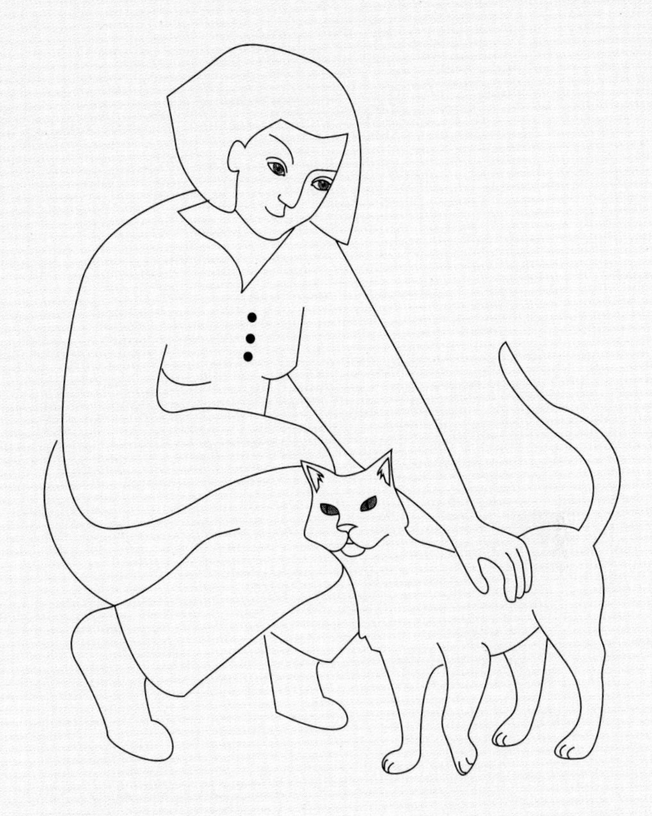

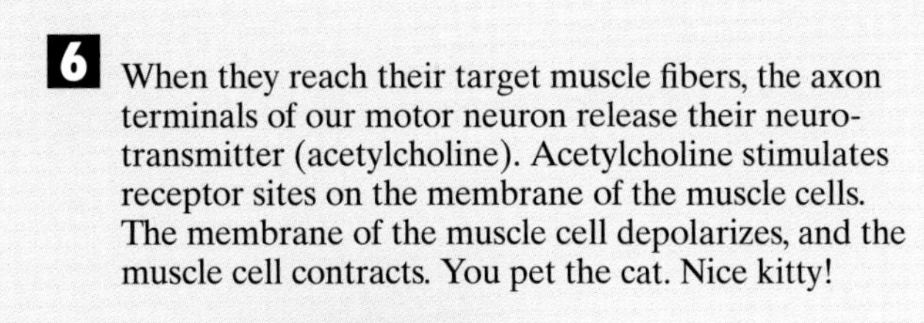

6 When they reach their target muscle fibers, the axon terminals of our motor neuron release their neurotransmitter (acetylcholine). Acetylcholine stimulates receptor sites on the membrane of the muscle cells. The membrane of the muscle cell depolarizes, and the muscle cell contracts. You pet the cat. Nice kitty!

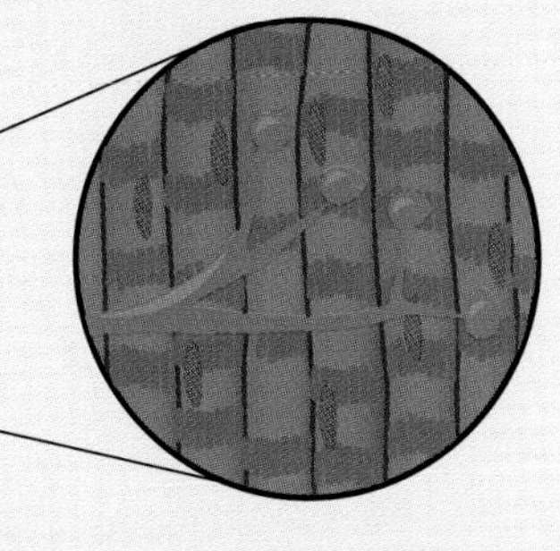

5 The axon of the motor neuron carries the nerve impulse to a target skeletal muscle. Skeletal muscles are made of many contractile muscle fibers. The nerve fiber meets its target muscle fibers at the *neuromuscular junction*.

Doing What Comes Naturally: The Spinal Reflexes

Automatic reflex responses to stimuli can involve two or more neurons that synapse in the spinal cord. The knee-jerk reflex is a good example of a monosynaptic (one-synapse) spinal reflex. Although this reflex does not directly involve the brain, the reflex itself may be exaggerated when there is brain damage.

1 The reflex is initiated by striking the patellar tendon with a hammer below the kneecap. Specialized stretch receptors located in the tendon, are stimulated, and they generate a nerve impulse in the sensory neuron.

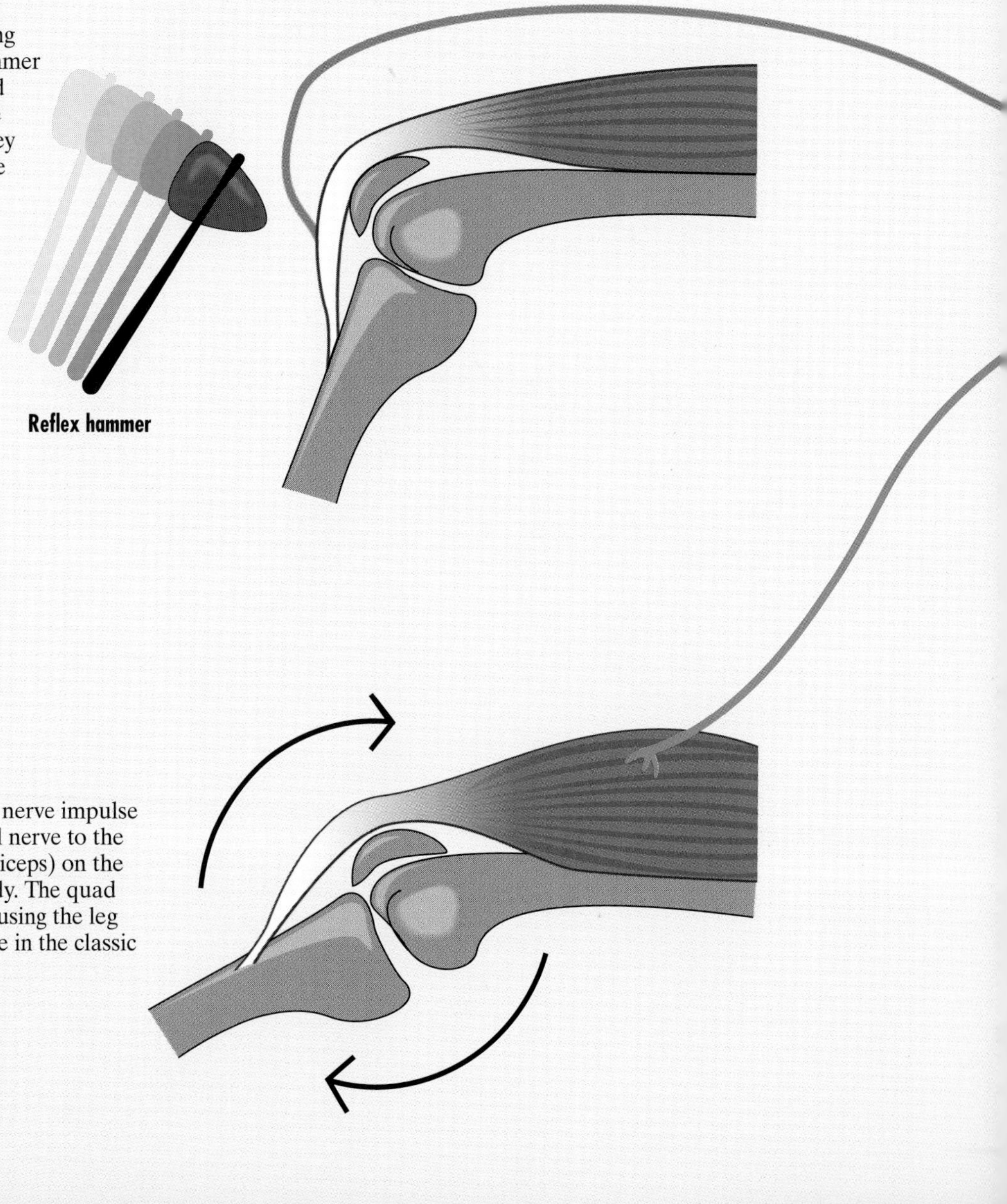

Reflex hammer

4 The motor neuron's nerve impulse travels via the spinal nerve to the thigh muscle (quadriceps) on the same side of the body. The quad muscle contracts, causing the leg to extend at the knee in the classic knee-jerk response.

2 The sensory nerve impulse travels to the spinal cord via the spinal nerve and its posterior (dorsal) root ganglion.

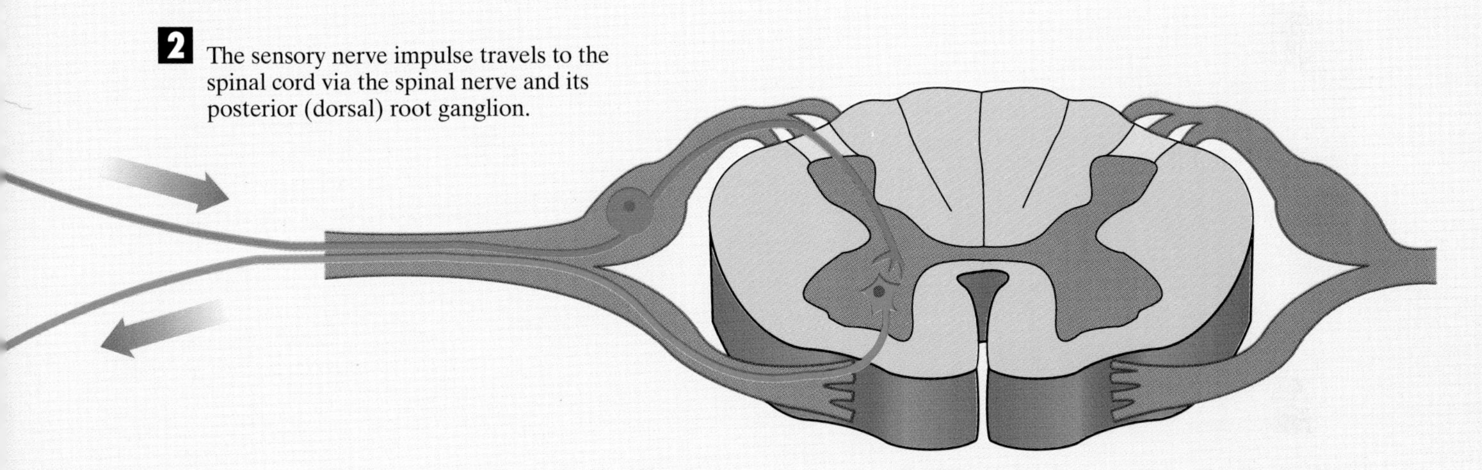

3 Within the butterfly-shaped gray matter of the spinal cord, the axon of the sensory neuron makes a synapse with the cell body of the motor neuron. A nerve impulse is generated in the motor neuron.

EXAGGERATED REFLEX It is known that some upper motor neurons (neurons bringing motor responses down from the brain to the spinal cord) can contribute to a baseline inhibitory effect on our lower motor neuron (shown in blue in the above illustration, with its cell body in the spinal gray matter). When there is a medical problem that destroys the upper motor neuron, its baseline inhibitory effect on the lower motor neuron is lost. When this happens, lower motor neurons that have lost their inhibitions are free to give exaggerated responses to stimuli. So, in cases of upper motor neuron illness, the knee-kerk reflex is exaggerated; this points to a problem higher in the nervous system.

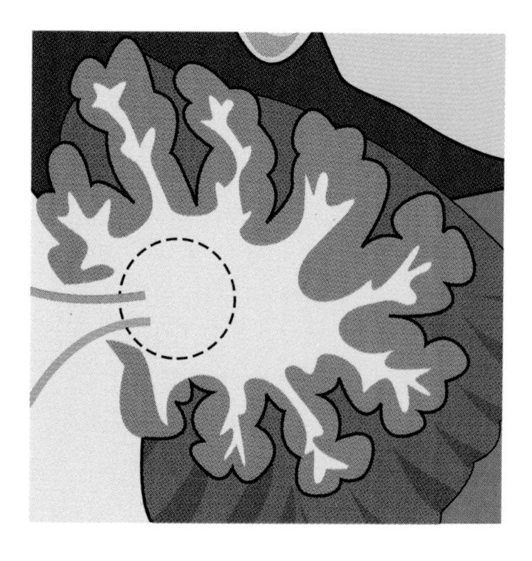

The Cerebellum
A Balance of Power

OUR BODIES ARE constantly doing subconscious things that our cerebral hemispheres don't need to think about. The popular subconscious functions—breathing, digestion, circulation—are well known because they are truly vital functions. But another realm of subconscious activity exists in the brain, and it gets much less publicity. It includes balance and equilibrium, posture, and coordination, and it is governed, in part, by the cerebellum.

When compared to the rest of the brain, the cerebellum looks like an annex. Its surface is wrinkled with ridges (*folia*), and its two hemispheres are separated by an elevation called the vermis (Latin for *worm*). Three trunks of white matter, the cerebellar peduncles, provide the only communication links between the cerebellum and the rest of the neural world. As a whole, the cerebellum is a rather isolated and homely place, and it doesn't even "think." So why is it important?

First of all, the cerebellum helps to balance the body. It consolidates input from position receptors in the limbs and head. Without consciousness, it knows where the body is, where it is going, how fast, and in what direction. It continually feeds its balancing instructions through neural pathways that help maintain posture and muscle tone.

Without the cerebellum, we could never keep on our toes or walk a straight line. For the athlete, ballet star, and steel worker alike, it is the cerebellum that balances, smooths out technique, and coordinates the limbs to create the "right moves."

The cerebellum appears to plan voluntary movements subconsciously before they are consciously executed by the cerebral hemispheres. Using a neural loop between the cerebral cortex and the cerebellum, the brain first subconsciously refines and plans body movements in the cerebellum, then consciously executes them via motor areas of the frontal lobes. In other words, before the cerebral cortex can execute the right moves, the cerebellum must first define exactly what "right" will mean. Only then can the actions of opposing muscles blend into one fluid motion, in the desired direction, at the desired time.

In its efforts to balance and coordinate the body, the cerebellum is helped by the basal ganglia, specialized islands of gray matter (nuclei) located deep within the white matter of the cerebral cortex. Together, the cerebellum and basal ganglia help the neural world to express its culture and soul—the poetic movements of dance, the skilled techniques of surgery, the smooth brush strokes of the artist—timing, precision, and grace.

Damage or disease in the cerebellum affects speed and quality of body movements, especially walking. Walking in a straight line becomes difficult, and people with cerebellar disease may need to lean on a wall or table for stability. There is also a characteristic wide-based stance and gait, because the body is more easily stabilized with its feet spaced widely apart.

Disease in the cerebellar hemispheres may cause problems in limb coordination (ataxia); decreased muscle tone (hypotonia); speech that is slowed, slurred, or fragmented (dysarthria); rapid involuntary eye movements (nystagmus); and a shaking of the limbs during voluntary movement (intention tremor). When only one cerebellar hemisphere is affected by disease or injury, the body will veer sideways toward the direction of the cerebellar problem—so a problem in the right cerebellar hemisphere will cause a person to veer to the right side.

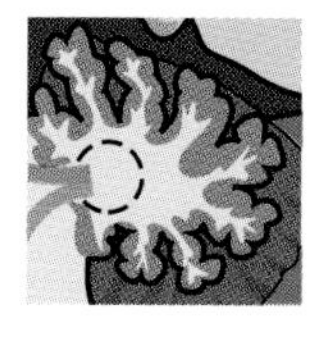

The midline vermis of the cerebellum can be damaged by alcohol abuse, resulting in alcoholic cerebellar degeneration. In this condition, neurons in the cortex of the cerebellar vermis degenerate. Symptoms include wide-based stance and gait, ataxia of the legs, and unstable posture of the trunk of the body.

The Cerebellum: Getting Your Bearings

The cerebellum helps to maintain the body's balance, muscle tone, and coordinated movements. The cerebellum lies below the occipital area of the cerebral hemispheres, behind the pons and medulla, and above the spinal cord.

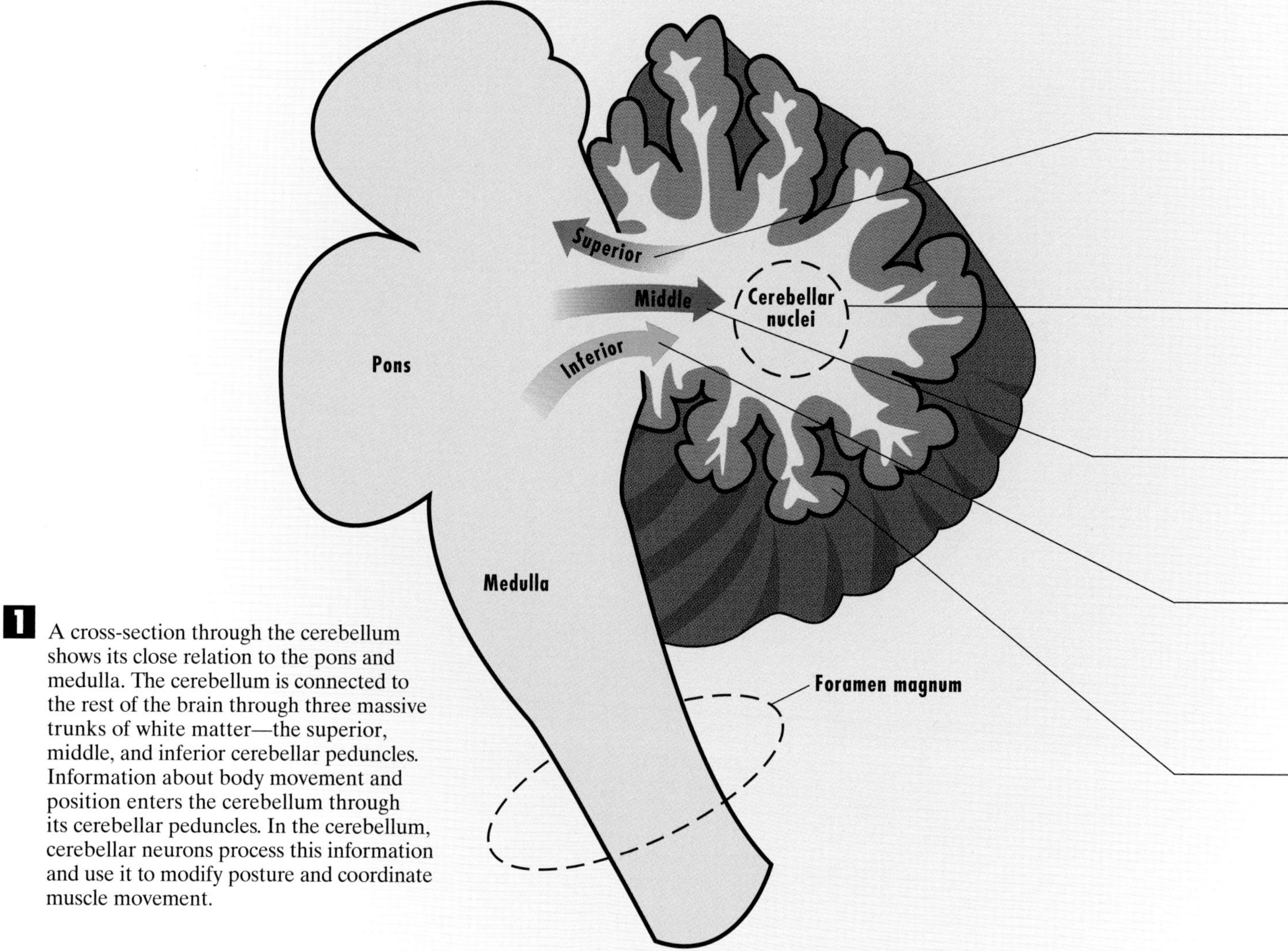

1 A cross-section through the cerebellum shows its close relation to the pons and medulla. The cerebellum is connected to the rest of the brain through three massive trunks of white matter—the superior, middle, and inferior cerebellar peduncles. Information about body movement and position enters the cerebellum through its cerebellar peduncles. In the cerebellum, cerebellar neurons process this information and use it to modify posture and coordinate muscle movement.

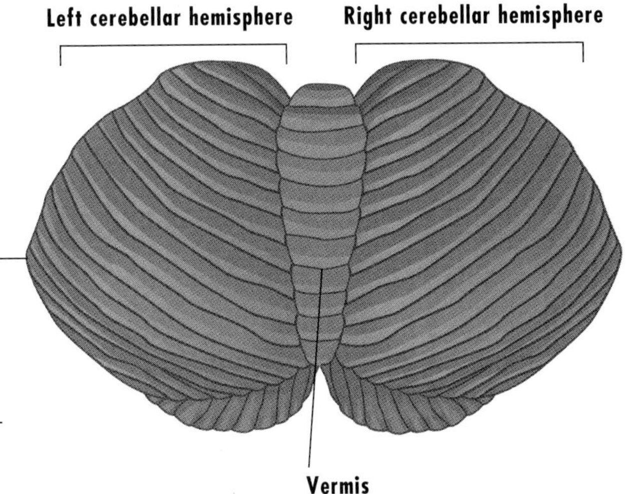

View of the Back of the Cerebellum

7 A view of the back of the brain (posterior surface) shows us the outside of the cerebellum. Like the cerebral cortex, the surface of the cerebellum has two hemispheres, the right and left cerebellar hemispheres. Instead of a midline fissure, the cerebellum has a midline swelling called the vermis. The surface of the cerebellum is covered with many tiny folds, the folia.

6 The *superior cerebellar peduncle* is primarily a conduit for outgoing (efferent) directions from the cerebellum. Most of its fibers originate in the cerebellar nuclei. Fibers that leave the cerebellum through the superior cerebellar peduncle ultimately go to brain structures that regulate muscle tone in the limbs and refine voluntary movements.

5 Below the cerebellar surface lie four pairs of *cerebellar nuclei.* The cerebellar nuclei receive input from the cerebellar cortex. They relay and mediate much of the communication between the cerebellar cortex and the peduncles.

4 The *middle cerebellar peduncle* is the largest. It brings information from the cerebral cortex to the cerebellum via connections in the pons. This incoming information is important to the cerebellum in coordinating movements of the extremities that require skill.

3 The *inferior cerebellar peduncle* connects the cerebellum to the medulla and channels mostly incoming (afferent) information. It brings data from the spinal cord concerning position of the body's limbs, and from the head—from position receptors in the facial muscles and from specialized motion receptors in the inner ear.

2 The cerebellum has an outside cortex of gray matter over a subsurface of white matter tracts. The gray matter is home for millions of neurons. *Purkinje cells*, the specialized neurons of the cerebellar cortex, have extensive dendrite branches. They can receive and process massive amounts of incoming information about the body's position and movement. Although the neurons of the cerebellum are always at work, their labors do not reach consciousness, and they do not "think" the way neurons in the cerebral cortex do.

Spatial Orientation and Posture: Knowing Where You Stand

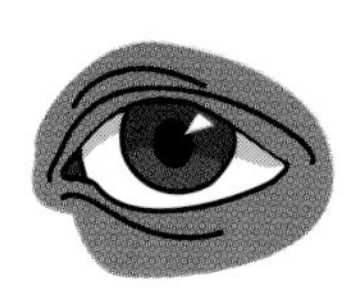

1 The brain needs to know the position and speed of the body as a whole. It must also know the position of each body limb. Some of this information comes through conscious visual pathways (sight) from the eyes to the occipital area of the cerebral cortex. These pathways do not involve the cerebellum, but they help us to see where we are.

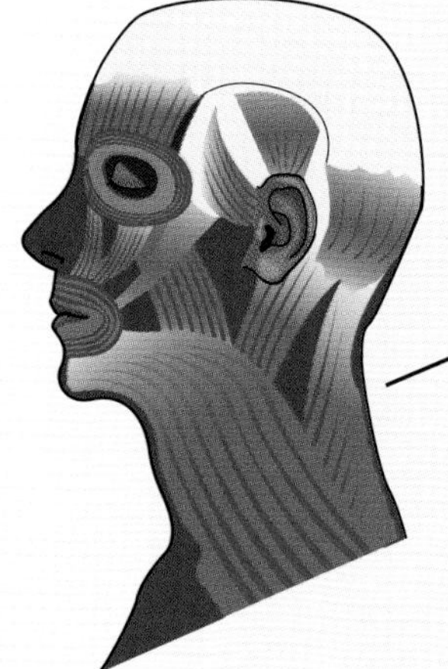

2 Some information about face position comes to the cerebellum by way of the trigeminocerebellar tract (via cranial nerve V) through the inferior cerebellar peduncle.

3 The vestibular system of the inner ear is an important source of information about head position. Receptors in the labyrinth of the inner ear are sensitive to all movements of the head, including acceleration and rotation. The fluid-filled tubes of the labyrinth's three semicircular canals respond to turning motions of the head. Other areas of the labyrinth respond to vertical jumping motion and to abrupt forward or backward movement.

4 Receptors in the vestibular system of the inner ear generate nerve impulses that are carried by the vestibular nerve (part of cranial nerve VIII). Information from the vestibular nerve eventually enters the cerebellum through the inferior cerebellar peduncle.

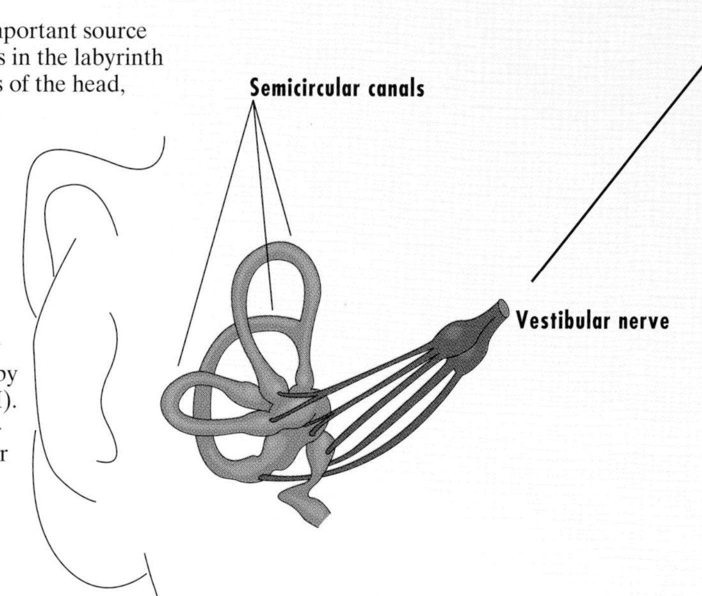

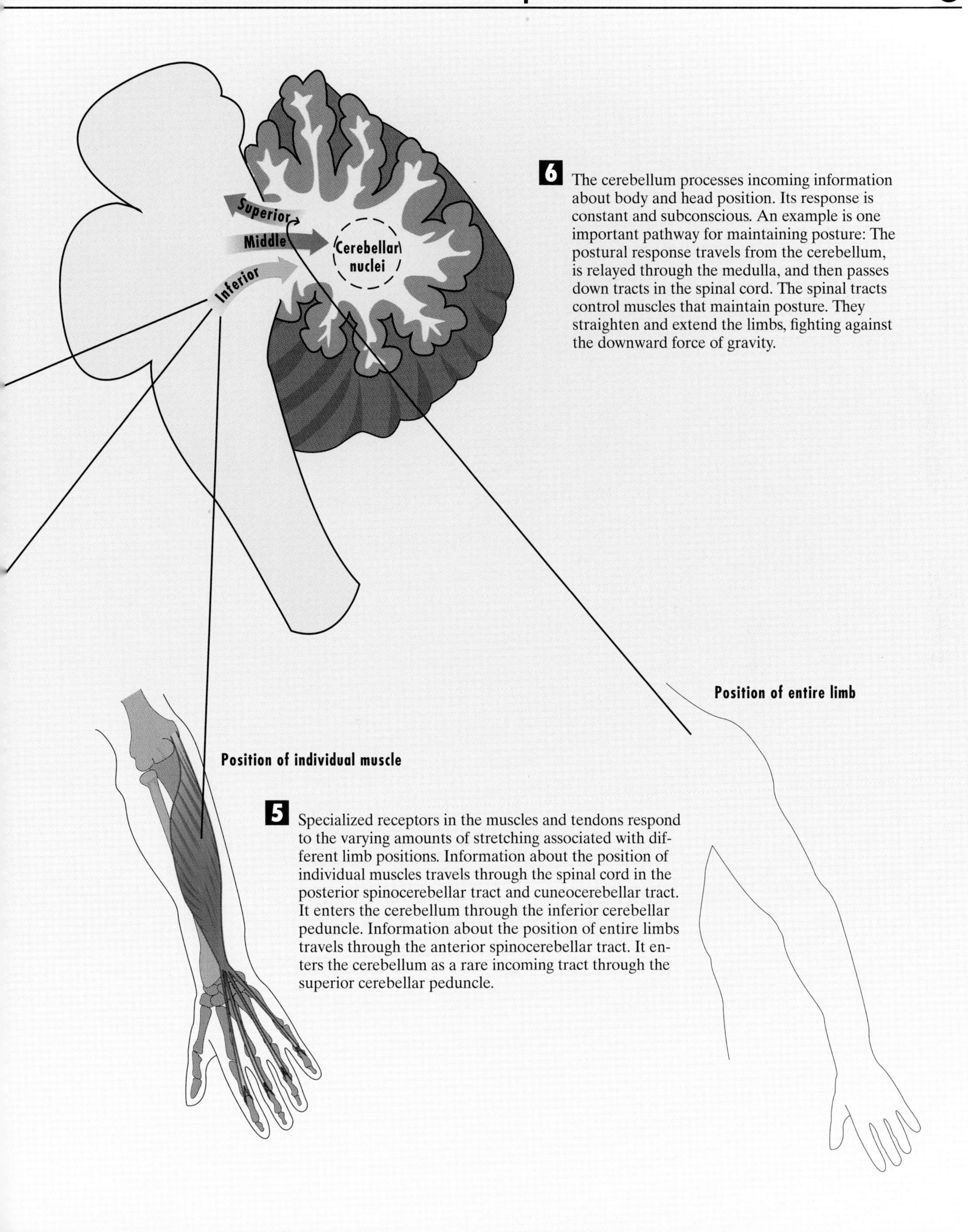

6 The cerebellum processes incoming information about body and head position. Its response is constant and subconscious. An example is one important pathway for maintaining posture: The postural response travels from the cerebellum, is relayed through the medulla, and then passes down tracts in the spinal cord. The spinal tracts control muscles that maintain posture. They straighten and extend the limbs, fighting against the downward force of gravity.

5 Specialized receptors in the muscles and tendons respond to the varying amounts of stretching associated with different limb positions. Information about the position of individual muscles travels through the spinal cord in the posterior spinocerebellar tract and cuneocerebellar tract. It enters the cerebellum through the inferior cerebellar peduncle. Information about the position of entire limbs travels through the anterior spinocerebellar tract. It enters the cerebellum as a rare incoming tract through the superior cerebellar peduncle.

Planning and Coordinating the Right Moves

1 The cerebellum subconsciously refines and plans commands for muscle movements before they are initiated by the cerebral cortex. One way that this is possible is through a pathway that loops from the cerebral cortex to the cerebellum, and then back again. The loop begins when the cerebral cortex sends information to the pons.

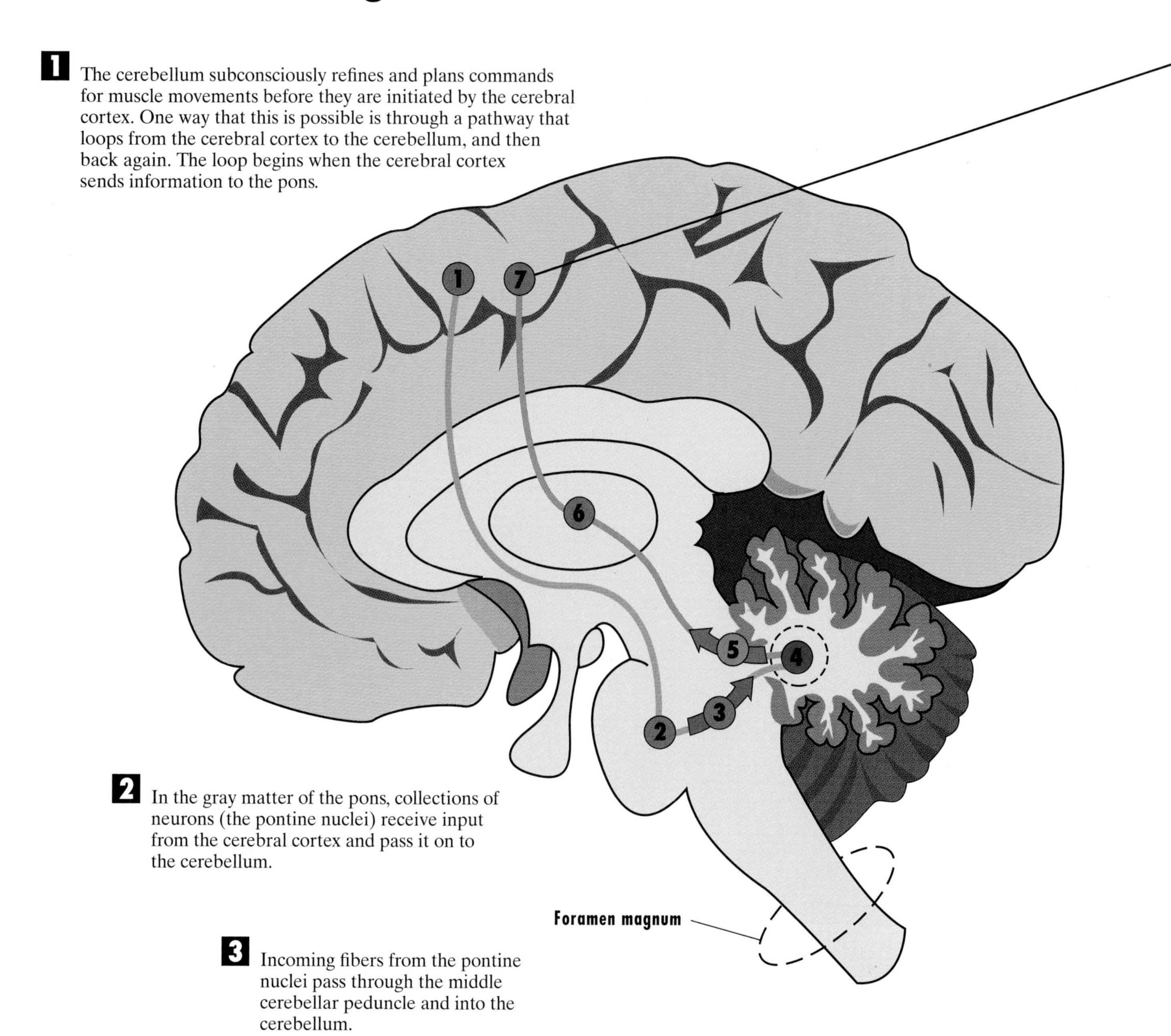

2 In the gray matter of the pons, collections of neurons (the pontine nuclei) receive input from the cerebral cortex and pass it on to the cerebellum.

3 Incoming fibers from the pontine nuclei pass through the middle cerebellar peduncle and into the cerebellum.

4 In the cerebellum, the incoming information is processed. The cerebellum formulates an outgoing response that is relayed through the cerebellar nuclei.

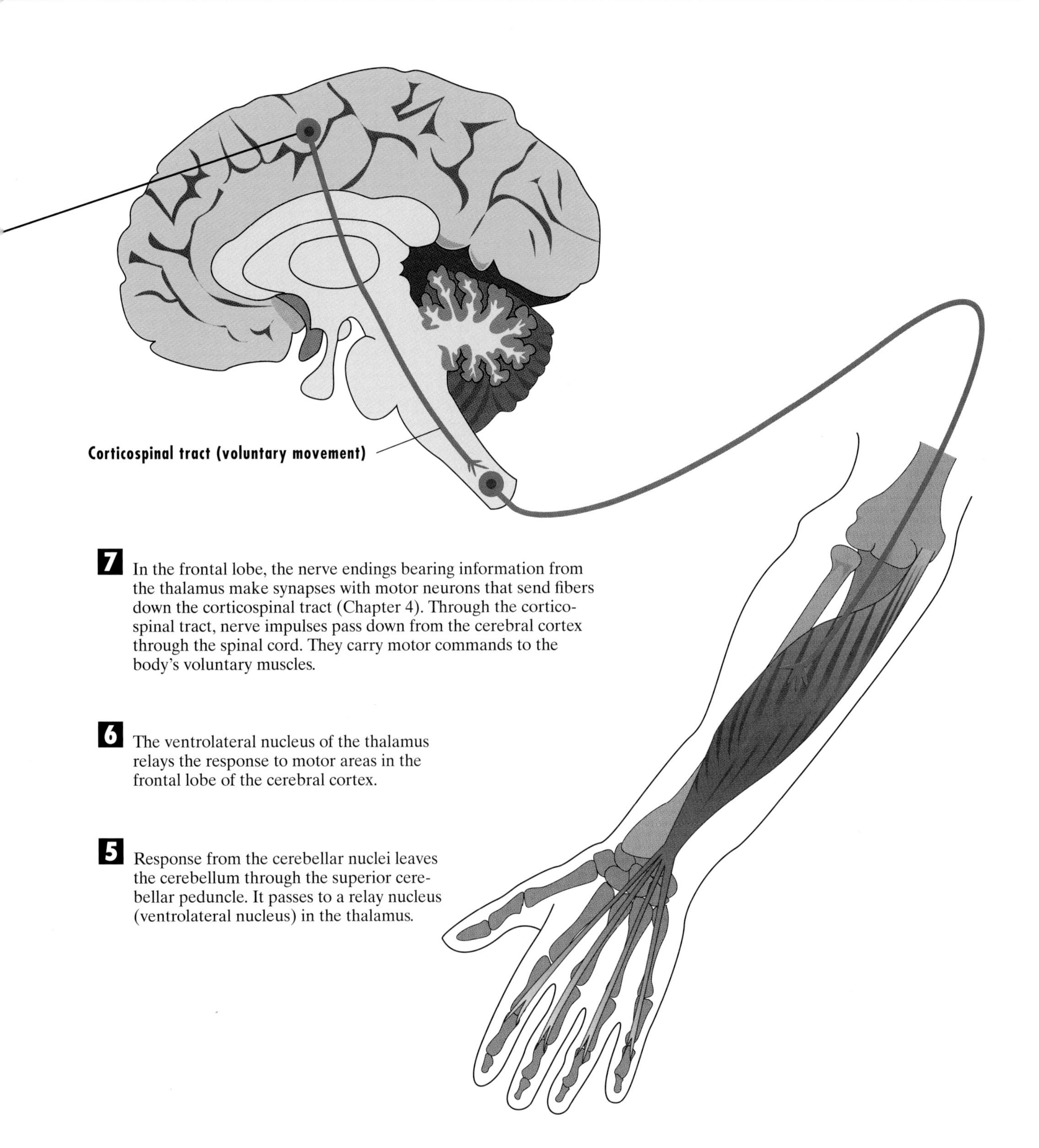

7 In the frontal lobe, the nerve endings bearing information from the thalamus make synapses with motor neurons that send fibers down the corticospinal tract (Chapter 4). Through the corticospinal tract, nerve impulses pass down from the cerebral cortex through the spinal cord. They carry motor commands to the body's voluntary muscles.

6 The ventrolateral nucleus of the thalamus relays the response to motor areas in the frontal lobe of the cerebral cortex.

5 Response from the cerebellar nuclei leaves the cerebellum through the superior cerebellar peduncle. It passes to a relay nucleus (ventrolateral nucleus) in the thalamus.

Vertigo and Parkinson's Disease: The World Spins and Shakes

1 Cerebellar disease is only rarely a cause of *vertigo*, the sensation that either the body or its surroundings is spinning or tilting. Vertigo can be accompanied by nausea and vomiting. Sometimes an anxious person may breathe abnormally fast (hyperventilate) and feel lightheaded, with more of a swaying than a spinning sensation. This may appear to be vertigo, but it is not true vertigo.

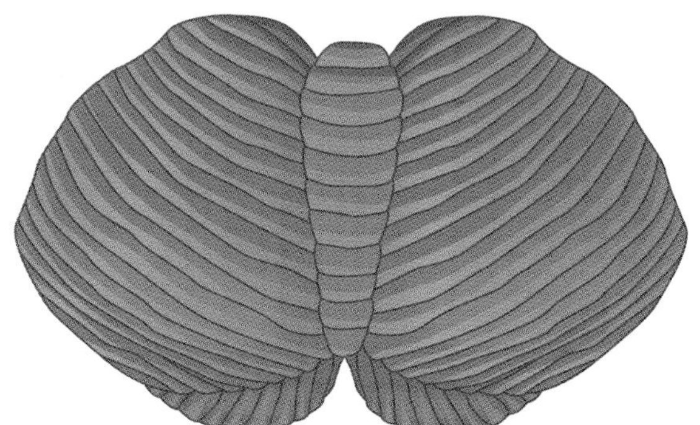

View of the Back of the Cerebellum

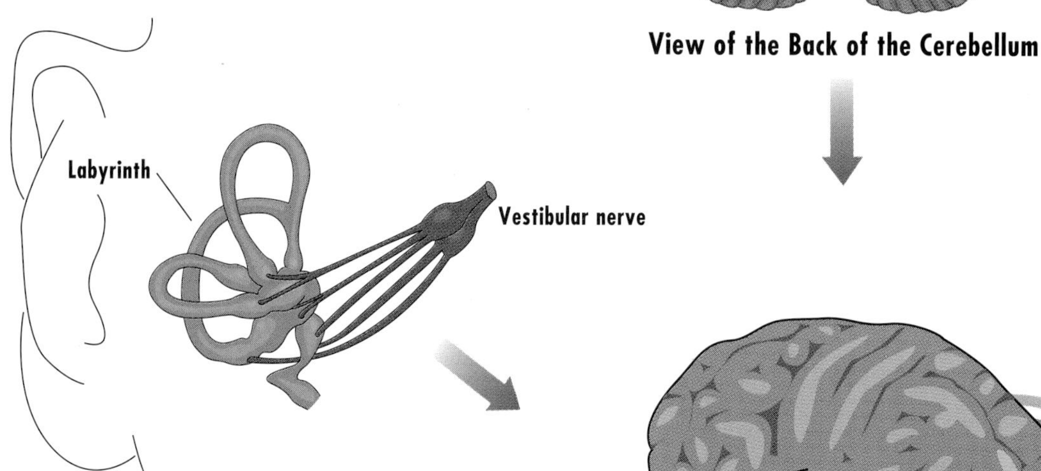

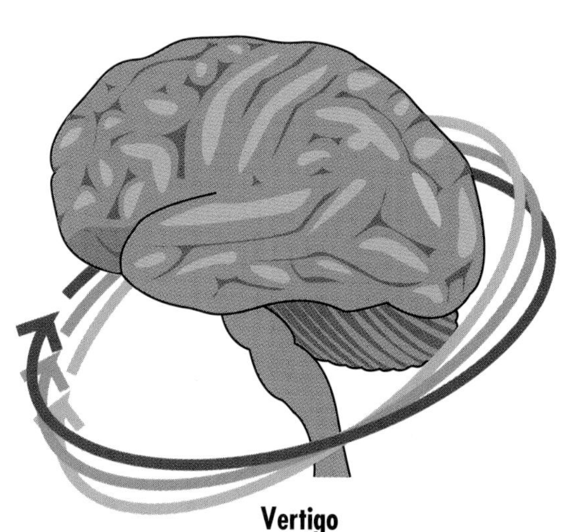

Vertigo

2 The most common cause of vertigo is a problem in the labyrinth of the inner ear—either in the labyrinth itself, its vestibular nerve, or its nuclei in the brain. In vestibular neuronitis, an infection affects the vestibular nerve and causes vertigo that can last for several days or weeks. In Ménière's disease, explosive attacks of vertigo usually occur together with deafness, buzzing in the ears (tinnitus), pallor, and vomiting. Ménière's disease can be treated by antihistamine drugs or, if necessary, by surgery of the inner ear.

THE BASAL GANGLIA.The basal ganglia are several islands of gray matter that lie embedded deep within the white matter of the cerebral hemispheres. Together with the cerebellum, the basal ganglia are activated before the voluntary corticospiinal pathways for movement come into play. They help plan and coordinate movement on a subconscious level. The amygdala, one of the basal ganglia, is located deep within the temporal lobe and has an important role in the limbic system (Chapter 8).

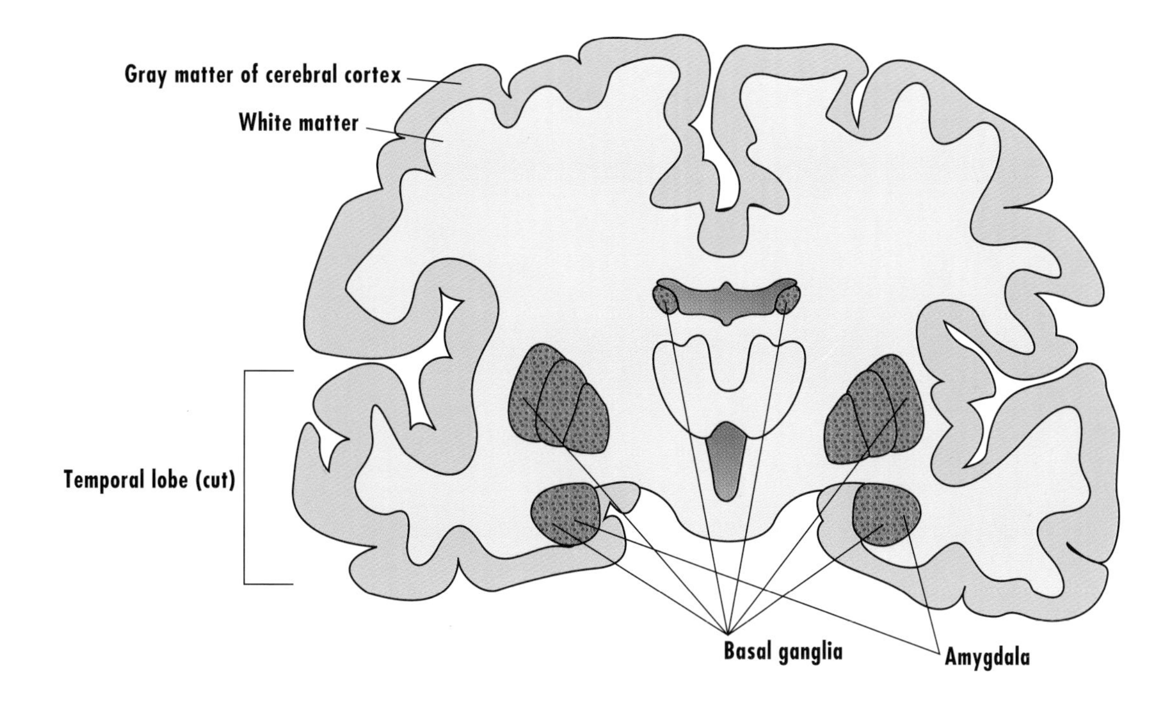

PARKINSON'S DISEASE In Parkinson's disease, one of the most well-known diseases of the basal ganglia, there is a tremor in limbs that are not moving (resting tremor). There is also rigidity, a tendency not to move parts of the body (poverty of movement), slowed movements, stooped posture, and a masklike facial expression. The gait is described as festinating—short, rapid steps, with the trunk of the body bent forward. Parkinson's disease is associated with a decrease in the neurotransmitter dopamine in parts of the basal ganglia, together with a degeneration of neurons. It is treated with drug therapy. A drug-induced syndrome that is similar to Parkinson's disease can occur in persons who have received large amounts of phenothiazines over a long period of time. Phenothiazines are drugs commonly used to treat schizophrenia.

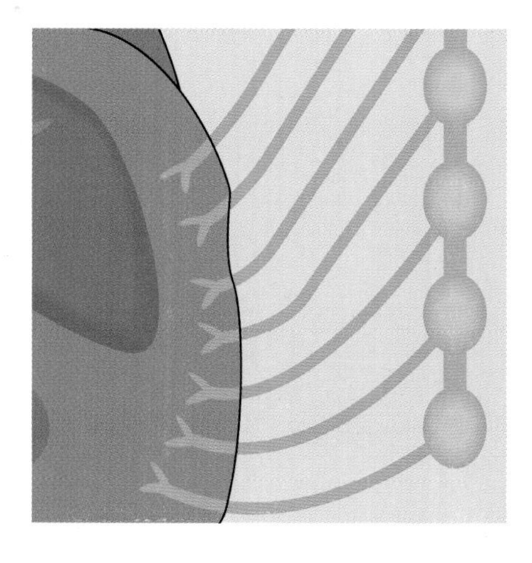

The Autonomic Nervous System
Essential Services

IN THE HUMAN world there are many essential services that we take for granted. Because most of us don't generate our own electricity or raise our own crops, we must depend on reliable people to do these things for us. And so it is in the brain.

Essential services for the neural world include respiration (breathing), digestion, and blood circulation. All of these come under the influence of a specialized organization of neurons called the *autonomic nervous system*, which is subdivided into sympathetic and parasympathetic parts.

Neurons located in the thoracic (chest) and lumbar (mid-back) regions of the spinal cord make up the *sympathetic* division of the autonomic nervous system. They send their impulses out through two chains of sympathetic ganglia, which run like strings of pearls on either side of the vertebral column. From neurons in the sympathetic ganglia, fibers project to blood vessels and sweat glands, and also to important internal organs such as the heart, lungs, stomach, intestines, and genitals. Sympathetic stimulation produces increased heart rate and stronger heart muscle contractions, constriction of blood vessels and increased blood pressure, dilation (opening up) of airways in the lungs, decreased movement of digestive organs; and "goose bumps" on the skin. In general, norepinephrine is the neurotransmitter at the nerve endings of sympathetic nerves.

Actions of the sympathetic nervous system are balanced by the second part of the autonomic nervous system, the *parasympathetic* division. Agents for the parasympathetic nervous system reside in selected cranial nerves (such as the vagus) and in the sacral (lower back) region of the spinal cord. Parasympathetic ganglia do not run in chains, but are located near the organs that they influence. Parasympathetic stimulation causes decreased heart rate and decreased strength of heart muscle contraction, dilation of blood vessels, constriction of air passages in the lungs, and increased movement of digestive organs. Acetylcholine is the parasympathetic neurotransmitter.

The autonomic nervous system oversees the body's vital functions through subconscious reflexes that balance its sympathetic and parasympathetic parts. Using the diplomacy of the autonomic network, the brain manipulates the organ systems on which it relies for life-sustaining food and oxygen. This frees the brain's neuron population to pursue their own vocations in the conscious services—sight, speech, hearing, thinking (association), emotion, and voluntary movement.

Brain and Heart: Neural Control of Circulation

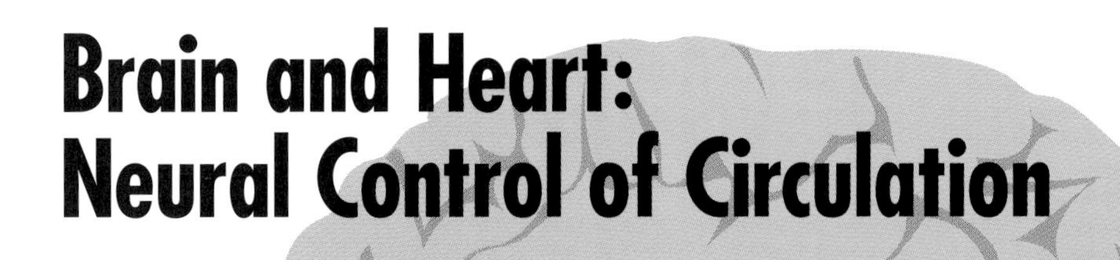

3 The vagus nerve (cranial nerve X) is the agent of the parasympathetic nervous system that makes contact with the SA node and AV node. Strong parasympathetic vagal activity can decrease the heart rate or even stop the heartbeat. If the vagus does stop the heartbeat for a few seconds, the heart will escape from vagal control and generate its own heartbeat, but at a slower rate of about 30 beats per minute. Parasympathetic stimulation can also decrease the strength of heart muscle contractions and decrease the heart's output by up to 50%.

2 The two chains of sympathetic ganglia, one on each side of the vertebral column, send nerve fibers that infiltrate the walls of the heart muscle. Sympathetic stimulation increases the heart rate and increases the strength of heart muscle contractions. The heart rate can jump to over 200 beats per minute, and the amount of blood pumped each minute can double or triple.

1 The heart can establish its own rhythm without any outside interference. The SA node (sinoatrial node), located in the right atrium, is the heart's pacemaker. It is made of self-excitatory cells that can generate impulses for heart muscle contractions at a rate of about 70 beats per minute. From the SA node, impulses pass to the AV node (atrioventricular node), and from the AV node to the heart muscle. If the AV system doesn't receive its expected input from the SA node, it can generate its own heart rhythm at 15–40 beats per minute. The parasympathetic nervous system sends fibers to both the SA and the AV nodes.

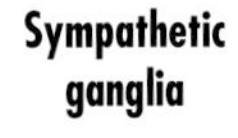

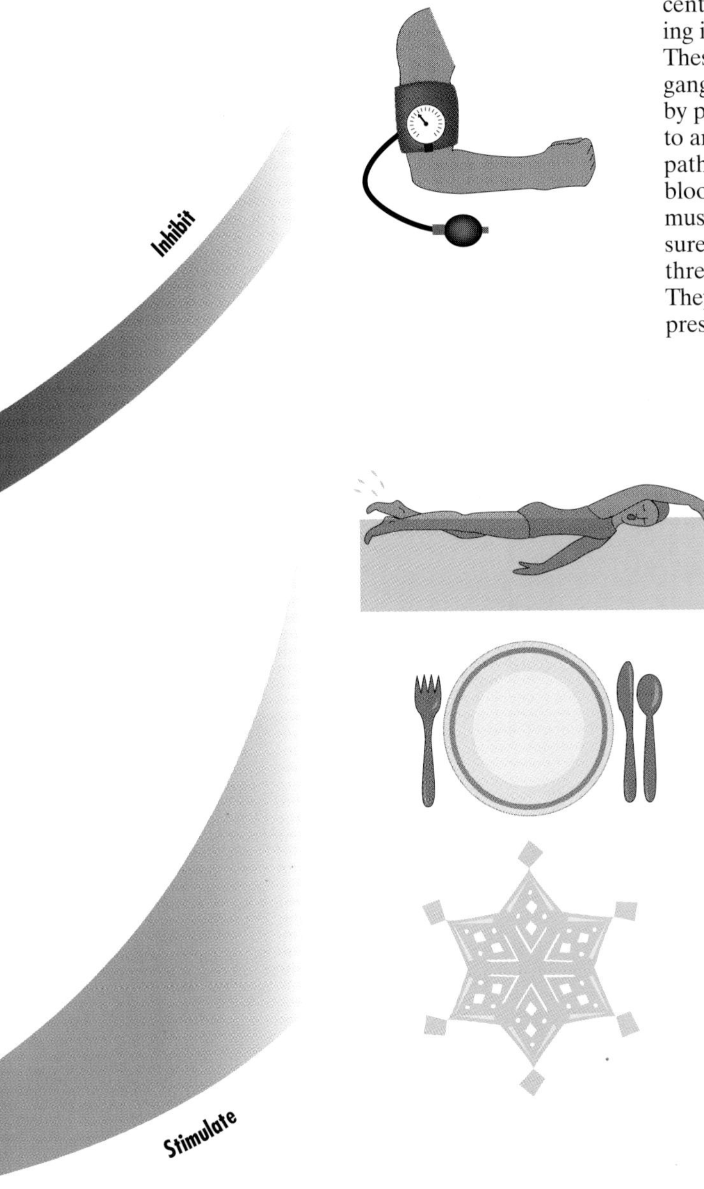

Sympathetic Brain Stem Centers and Blood Pressure Control Sympathetic centers in the brain stem help to maintain a normal blood pressure by sending impulses to the heart and to the muscles in the walls of blood vessels. These impulses travel down the spinal cord and pass through the sympathetic ganglia. Under normal conditions, if blood pressure gets too high, it is sensed by pressure receptors in the body's blood vessels. This information is relayed to an area in the brain stem that will *inhibit* (shut down) the brain stem sympathetic centers. Inhibition of the brain stem sympathetic center causes the blood pressure to drop by decreasing the heart's activity and relaxing the muscles in the walls of blood vessels. In people with chronic high blood pressure (hypertension), pressure receptors in the blood vessels may have their thresholds reset so that they begin to read higher blood pressures as normal. They can still respond to an increase in blood pressure, but it takes a higher pressure level to stimulate them.

Sympathetic Stimulations and Angina The sympathetic nervous system can be activated by eating, exercise, and exposure to cold. Sympathetic stimulation increases both the heart rate and the strength of heart muscle contractions, which increases the workload on the heart. With increased workload, the coronary arteries must supply more blood to the busy heart muscle. But if there is coronary artery disease, the coronary blood supply may not be able to meet the increased demands of the heart. This can trigger the chest pain of angina.

Stimulate

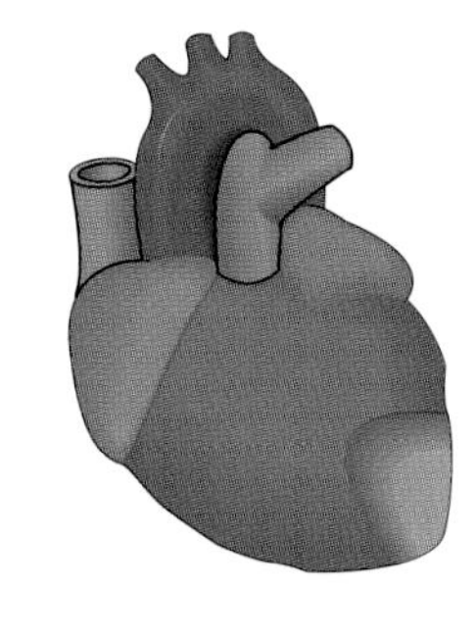

Sympathetic Reflexes and Heart Attack When a coronary artery is blocked and a person suffers a heart attack (myocardial infarction), sympathetic reflexes may be triggered to respond to the heart's decreased ability to pump blood. This sympathetic stimulation increases the "irritability" of the heart and increases the risk of developing a dangerously abnormal heart rhythm called ventricular fibrillation, whereby the chaotic rhythm prevents the heart muscle from contracting effectively, causing cardiac arrest.

Brain and Lungs: Neural Control of Breathing

1 We need to take in oxygen to metabolize (burn) the food we eat. We also need to eliminate carbon dioxide, a waste product that is made by our body cells. Breathing allows our blood to absorb oxygen and eliminate carbon dioxide. During normal "quiet" breathing at rest, the body inhales by actively expanding the chest to take air into the lungs. After inhaling, the natural stiffness of the chest muscles and lungs makes them recoil automatically to exhale air. So, at rest, exhaling is a passive act that doesn't need muscular effort.

2 Quiet breathing at rest has a natural rhythm that is regulated subconsciously by an inspiratory center in the medulla of the brain. The rhythm of breathing is controlled by a group of neurons in the medulla called the *dorsal respiratory group*. From the dorsal respiratory group, impulses pass down to stimulate contractions of the diaphragm and the intercostal muscles between the ribs. This expands the chest, creating a negative pressure that draws air into the lungs. When the dorsal respiratory group rhythmically shuts off, the chest muscles relax and the air is passively exhaled.

3 Near the dorsal respiratory group is another collection of neurons called the *ventral respiratory group*. These neurons play no part in quiet breathing at rest. They are activated only when the respiratory system goes into overdrive, as in exercise.

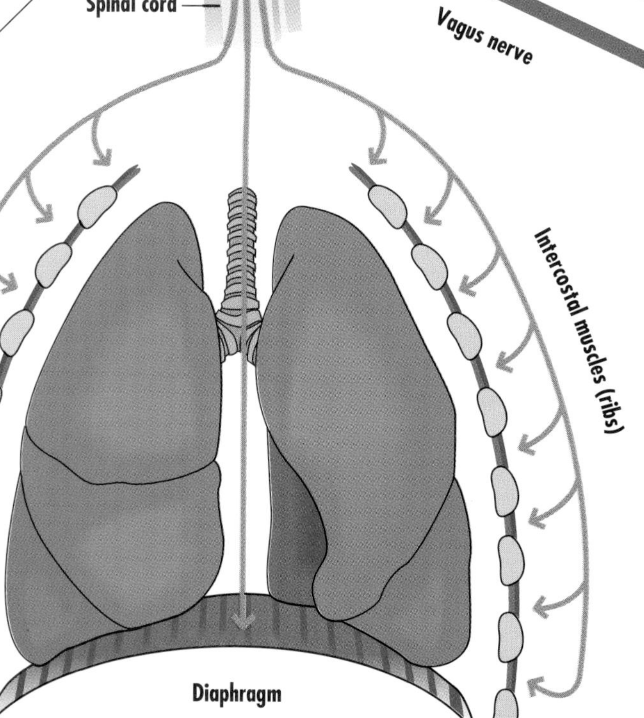

4 High in the upper pons the *pneumotaxic center* regulates the length of each breath. It shuts off the dorsal respiratory group when an inhaled breath has lasted long enough.

8 Because the cerebral cortex has some control over breathing activity, it is possible to consciously hold your breath. In this case, the nerve impulse doesn't go to the lungs through the respiratory center in the medulla. Rather, it goes down the usual paths for voluntary muscle control—down the corticospinal tract (see Chapter 4) to spinal nerves that control the respiratory muscles.

7 Because the cerebrospinal fluid (CSF) has its origin in blood (see Chapter 3), the amount of carbon dioxide in CSF reflects the amount of carbon dioxide in the bloodstream. Chemoreceptors on the surface of the brain in the area of the medulla's respiratory center are stimulated by excess carbon dioxide in the CSF, and they can directly trigger the respiratory center to increase breathing activity.

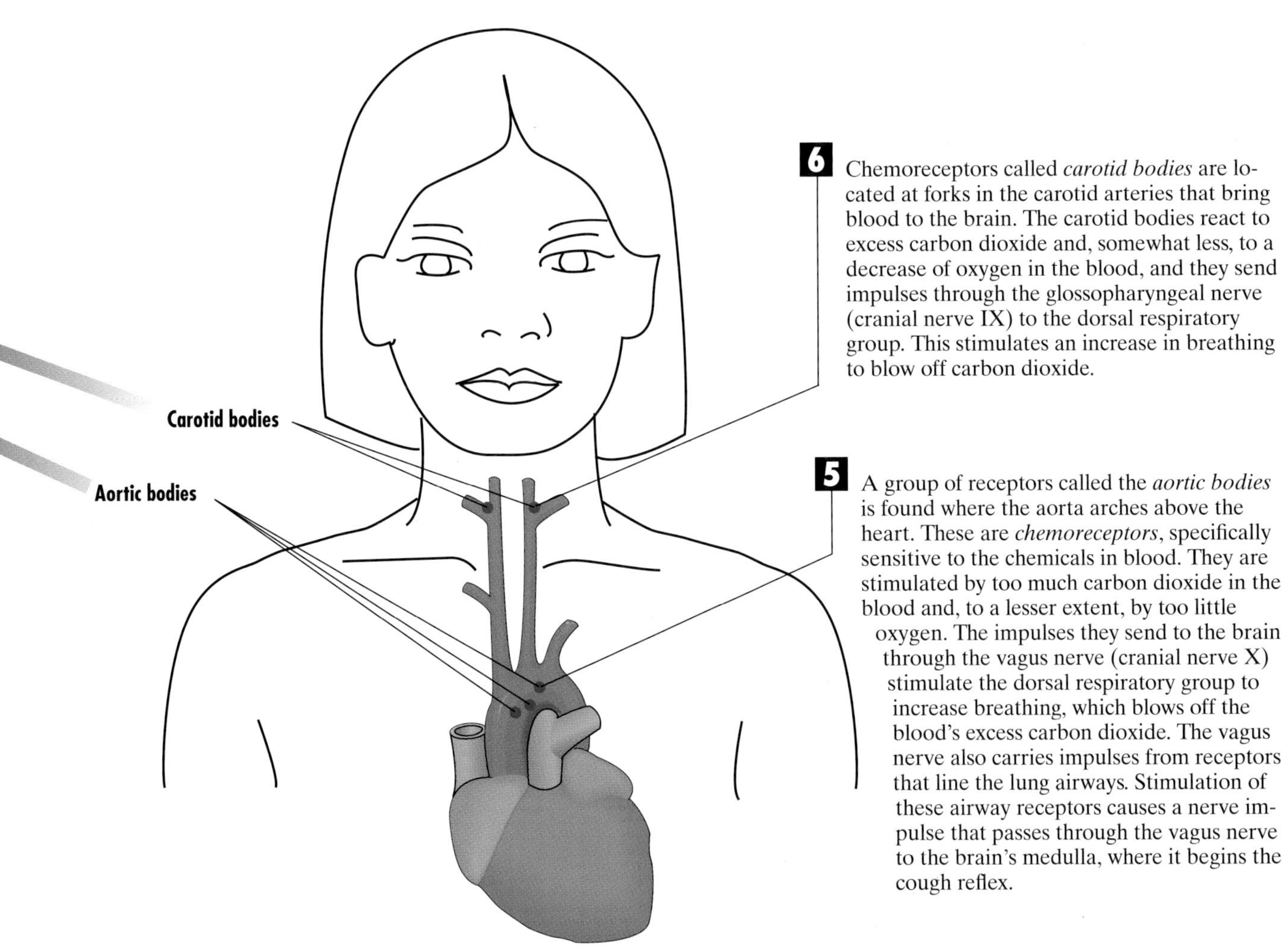

6 Chemoreceptors called *carotid bodies* are located at forks in the carotid arteries that bring blood to the brain. The carotid bodies react to excess carbon dioxide and, somewhat less, to a decrease of oxygen in the blood, and they send impulses through the glossopharyngeal nerve (cranial nerve IX) to the dorsal respiratory group. This stimulates an increase in breathing to blow off carbon dioxide.

5 A group of receptors called the *aortic bodies* is found where the aorta arches above the heart. These are *chemoreceptors*, specifically sensitive to the chemicals in blood. They are stimulated by too much carbon dioxide in the blood and, to a lesser extent, by too little oxygen. The impulses they send to the brain through the vagus nerve (cranial nerve X) stimulate the dorsal respiratory group to increase breathing, which blows off the blood's excess carbon dioxide. The vagus nerve also carries impulses from receptors that line the lung airways. Stimulation of these airway receptors causes a nerve impulse that passes through the vagus nerve to the brain's medulla, where it begins the cough reflex.

Brain and Stomach: Neural Control of Digestion

1 Through parasympathetic activity, the brain can stimulate the digestive organs. The stomach is a good example. The sight, smell, and taste sensations of food reach their respective sensation areas in the occipital, frontal and/or temporal, and parietal lobes of the cerebral cortex. Nerve impulses from the cerebral cortex activate a vagal center in the medulla.

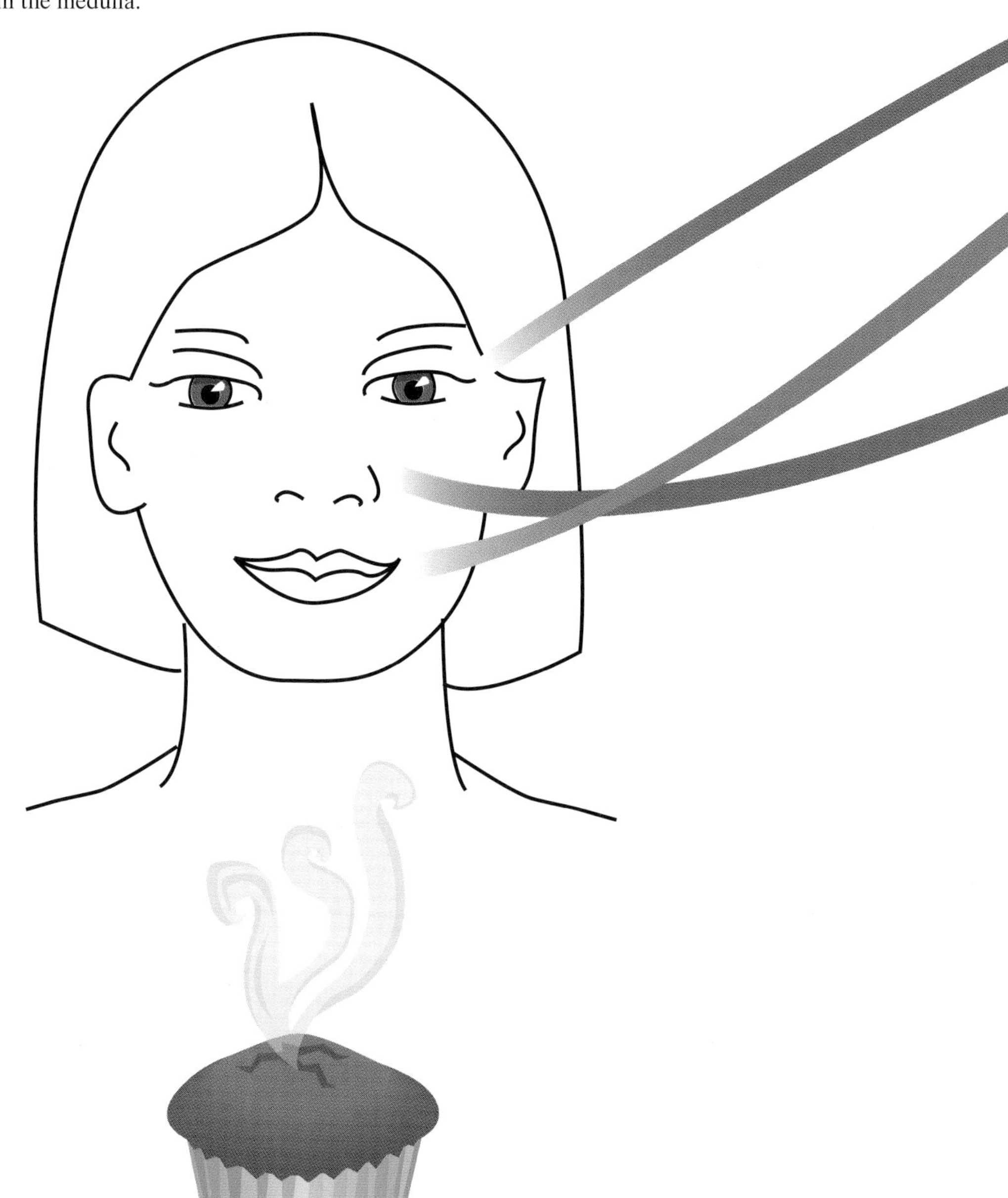

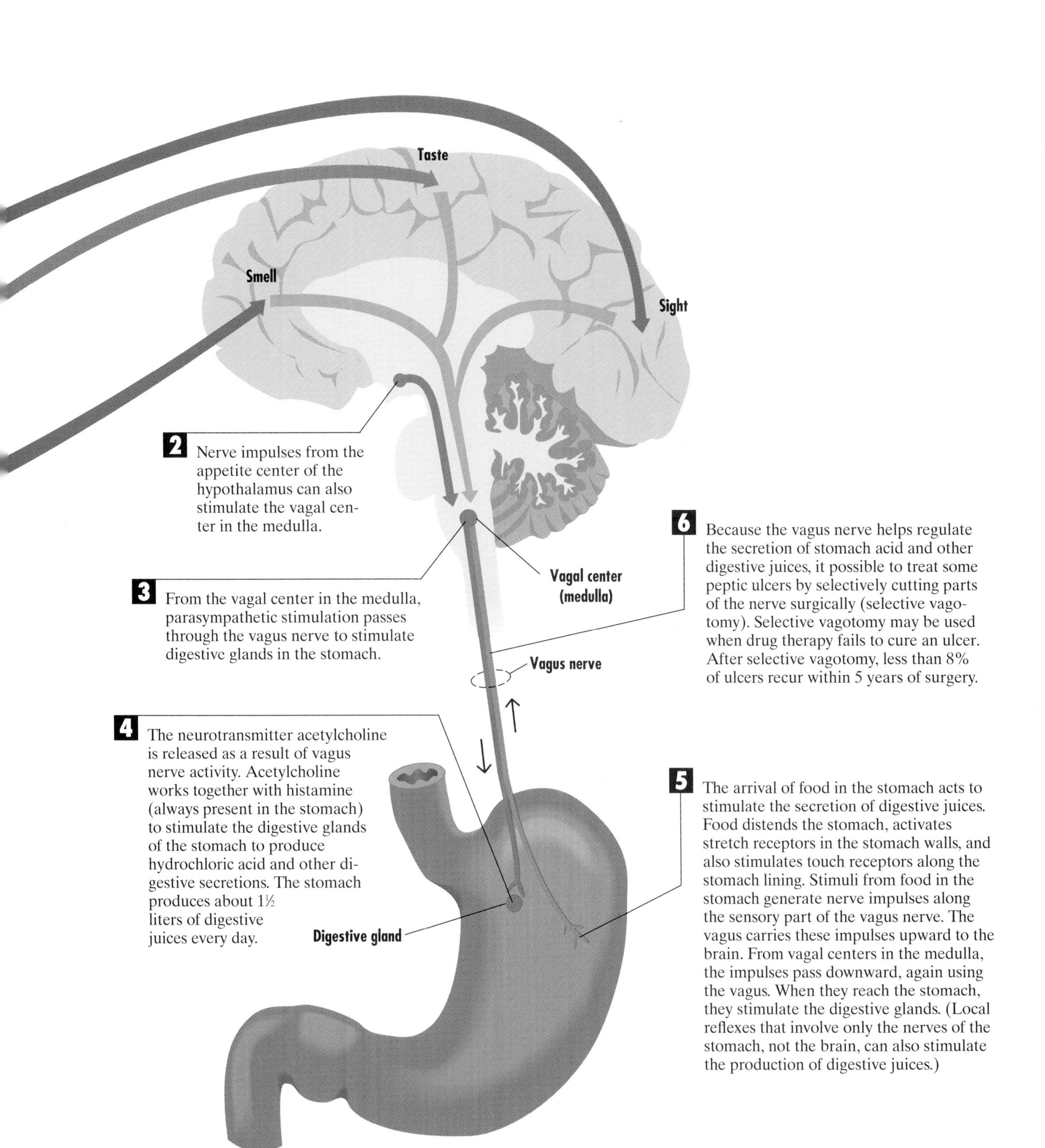

2 Nerve impulses from the appetite center of the hypothalamus can also stimulate the vagal center in the medulla.

3 From the vagal center in the medulla, parasympathetic stimulation passes through the vagus nerve to stimulate digestive glands in the stomach.

4 The neurotransmitter acetylcholine is released as a result of vagus nerve activity. Acetylcholine works together with histamine (always present in the stomach) to stimulate the digestive glands of the stomach to produce hydrochloric acid and other digestive secretions. The stomach produces about 1½ liters of digestive juices every day.

5 The arrival of food in the stomach acts to stimulate the secretion of digestive juices. Food distends the stomach, activates stretch receptors in the stomach walls, and also stimulates touch receptors along the stomach lining. Stimuli from food in the stomach generate nerve impulses along the sensory part of the vagus nerve. The vagus carries these impulses upward to the brain. From vagal centers in the medulla, the impulses pass downward, again using the vagus. When they reach the stomach, they stimulate the digestive glands. (Local reflexes that involve only the nerves of the stomach, not the brain, can also stimulate the production of digestive juices.)

6 Because the vagus nerve helps regulate the secretion of stomach acid and other digestive juices, it possible to treat some peptic ulcers by selectively cutting parts of the nerve surgically (selective vagotomy). Selective vagotomy may be used when drug therapy fails to cure an ulcer. After selective vagotomy, less than 8% of ulcers recur within 5 years of surgery.

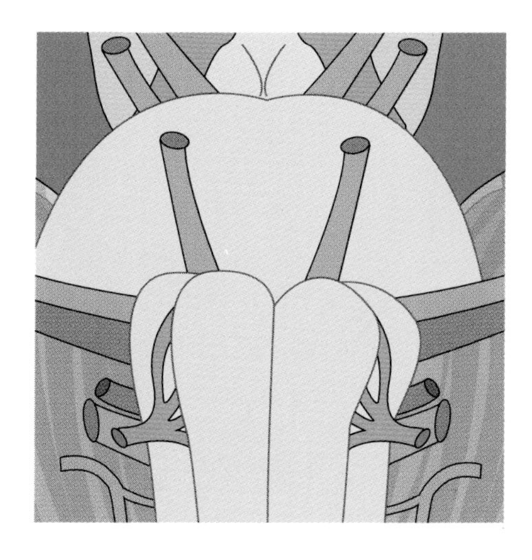

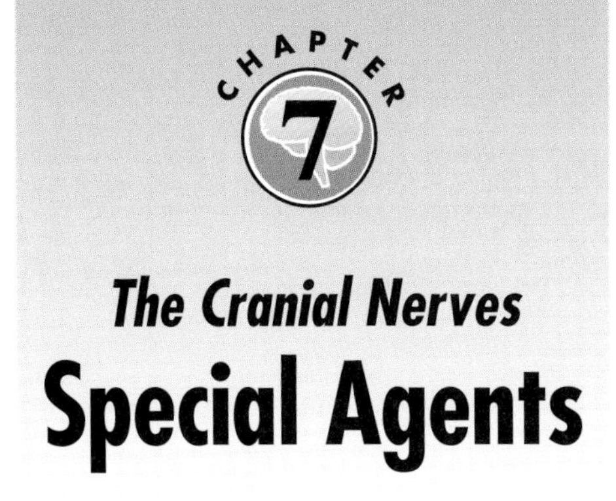

The Cranial Nerves
Special Agents

THE BRAIN, like most human governments, knows the power of the media, so it constantly monitors incoming information from the spinal nerves—touch, pain, pressure, and body position. But when vital "intelligence" information is needed, the brain, like human governments, relies on its own agents to gather data quickly and precisely. This is one function of the cranial nerves.

There are 12 pairs of cranial nerves, all linking the brain directly to important areas outside the skull. They may not seem familiar as a group, but individually they are well known. They include agents for four of the five senses: smell (olfactory nerves), sight (optic nerves), hearing (cochlear nerves), and taste (facial and glossopharyngeal nerves). The trigeminal nerve also receives touch sensations from all areas of the face, while the vagus keeps the brain in contact with the respiratory and digestive organs (Chapter 6). In practical terms, the cranial nerves warn the brain of all types of danger and participate in reflexes that make us cough, squint, sneeze, and blink.

Yet the cranial nerves have more than a sensory function. Like true and reliable agents, the cranial nerves can implement the brain's motor directives swiftly, using their own channels that lie outside the usual spinal motor pathways. They can turn and focus the eyes and regulate the size of the pupil. They can even turn the whole head when necessary. They can move the tongue and vocal cords to let us speak, and they can move the facial muscles to let us grimace and glare. They let us swallow hard and they let us spit.

Headquarters for most of the cranial nerves lie in the brain's cranial nerve nuclei. The cranial nerve nuclei are separate specialized populations of neurons within the brain that mediate the brain's communication with the cranial nerves. They mediate activities that are conscious (like hearing and taste) as well as those that are subconscious (like the pupil's response to light). The vestibular nuclei (cranial nerve VIII) detect head movements and have an intimate relationship with the cerebellum, while the nuclei of the vagus (cranial nerve X) have an important role in the parasympathetic nervous system (Chapter 6).

We will begin with an overview of all 12 cranial nerves, then focus on the pathways for sight and hearing. We will end our tour with a look at how several cranial nerves can coordinate their activities to produce the miracle of human speech.

The Cranial Nerves: Special Agents with Special Functions

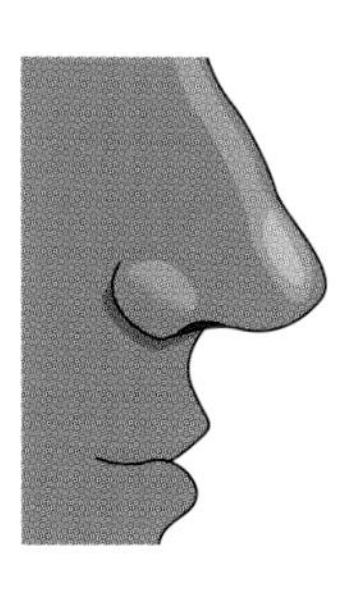

Olfactory Nerve (Cranial Nerve I) The thin fibers of the olfactory nerve originate in 100 million smell receptors on the roof of the nasal cavity. Olfactory nerve fibers carry information about environmental smells to the cerebral cortex and to the limbic system (Chapter 8), the seat of emotion.

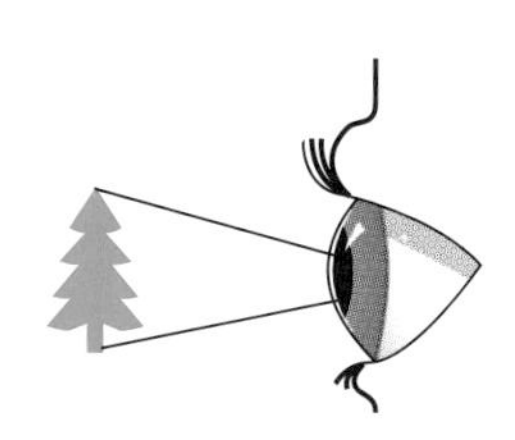

Optic Nerve (II) The optic nerve carries impulses for sight from the retina (at the back of the eye) to the occipital lobe of the cerebral cortex.

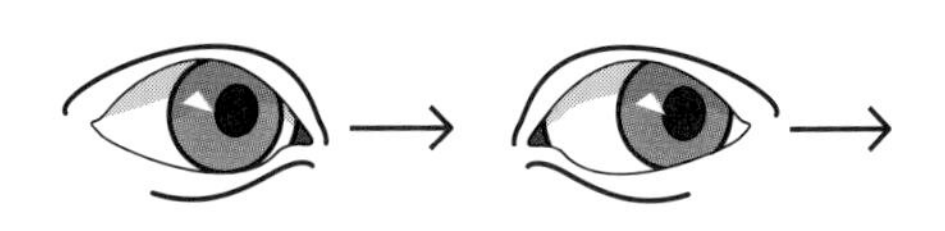

Cranial Nerves III, IV, and VI The oculomotor (III), trochlear (IV), and abducens (VI) cranial nerves control the muscles that move the eyeball in its socket. The oculomotor nerve also carries parasympathetic fibers that control the size of the pupils.

Oculomotor (III)

Trochlear (IV)

Abducens (VI)

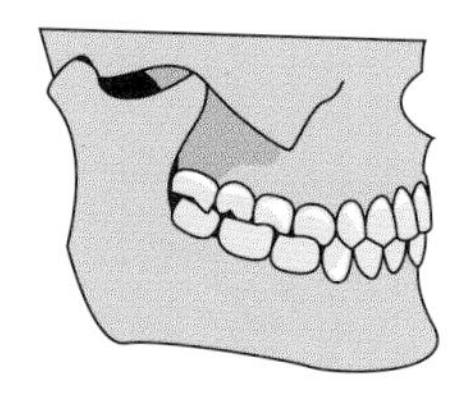

Trigeminal Nerve (V) The trigeminal nerve carries sensation from the skin of the face, from the cornea of the eye, and from the teeth. It carries the pain of toothaches and of temporomandibular joint dysfunction. Its motor portion controls the jaw muscles responsible for chewing movements.

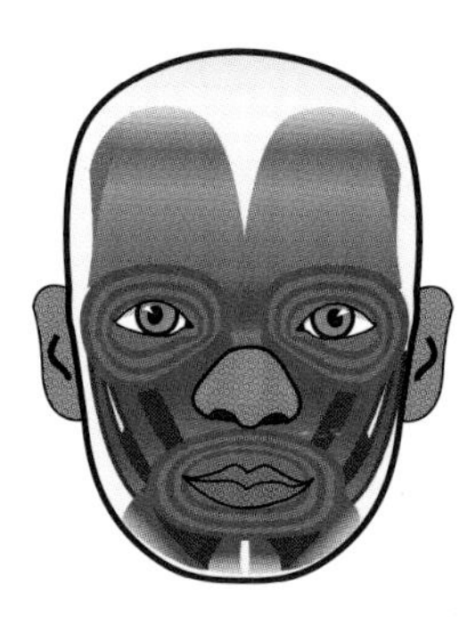

Facial Nerve (VII) The facial nerve controls the muscles of facial expression. It allows us to smile, frown, or show an expressionless "poker face." Paralysis of the right or left facial nerve causes a drooping of one side of the face (Bell's palsy). The facial nerve also carries taste from the front portion of the tongue and controls some of the salivary glands that make saliva.

Acoustic Nerve (VIII)
The acoustic nerve is also known as the auditory or vestibulocochlear nerve (emphasizing both of its functions). The vestibular portion arises from the labyrinth of the inner ear and carries sensory impulses that detect head position and movement (Chapter 5). The cochlear portion carries impulses for the sense of hearing.

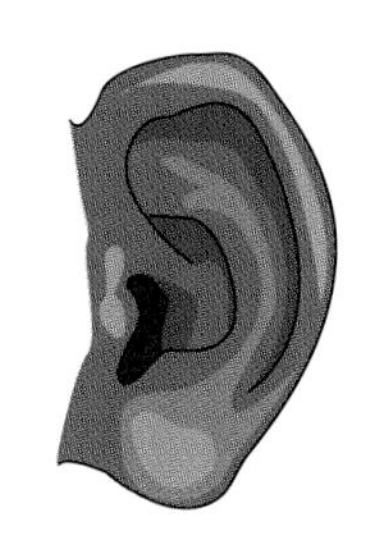

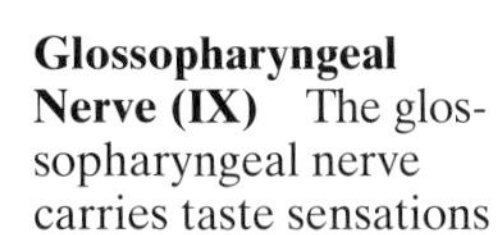

Glossopharyngeal Nerve (IX) The glossopharyngeal nerve carries taste sensations from the back portion of the tongue. The nerve also carries pain and touch sensations—including sore throat pain—from the throat. The motor portion of this nerve controls a salivary gland in the cheek and muscles in the pharynx. A specialized part of the glossopharyngeal nerve also carries sensation from the carotid bodies, receptors that help regulate breathing (Chapter 6).

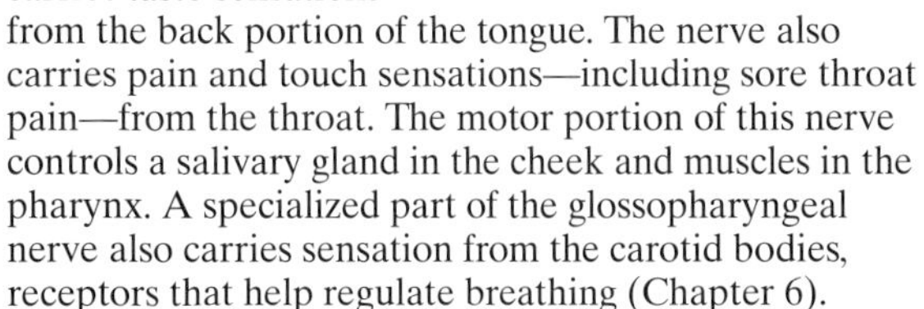

Vagus Nerve (X)
We have already seen the vagus as an active player in the parasympathetic regulation of vital bodily functions like breathing, digestion, and control of the heart. Two branches of the vagus, called the right and left recurrent laryngeal nerves, control the vocal cords on the right and left side of the neck.

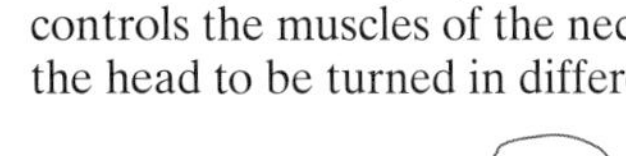

Accessory Nerve (XI) The accessory nerve controls the muscles of the neck that allow the head to be turned in different directions.

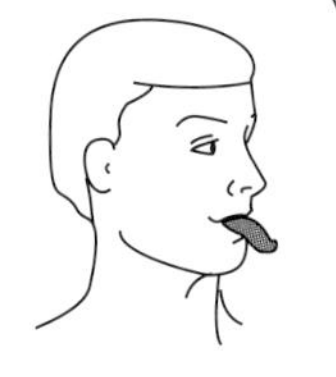

Hypoglossal Nerve (XII)
The hypoglossal nerve controls the tongue muscles.

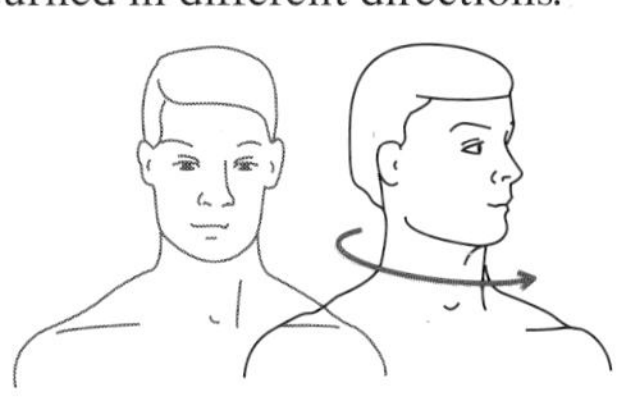

Sight: From the Eye to the Cortex

1 To follow the pathways for sight, we imagine a section of brain lying in a plane that stretches from the eyes to the occipital lobe (shown below and at right). The pathways begin at the retina, a light-sensitive layer at the back of the eyes. The retina is lined by specialized light receptors: 100 million rods to sense low light, and 7 million cones for higher resolution and color vision. Rods and cones synapse with a series of cells that finally form the assembled axons of the optic nerve.

2 The arrangement of axons in the optic nerve is not haphazard. Axons from the part of the retina nearest the nose (the nasal or medial part) travel in the portion of the optic nerve closest to the midline, while axons from the part of the retina nearest the temples (the temporal or lateral part) travel in the portion of the optic nerve closest to the sides of the head.

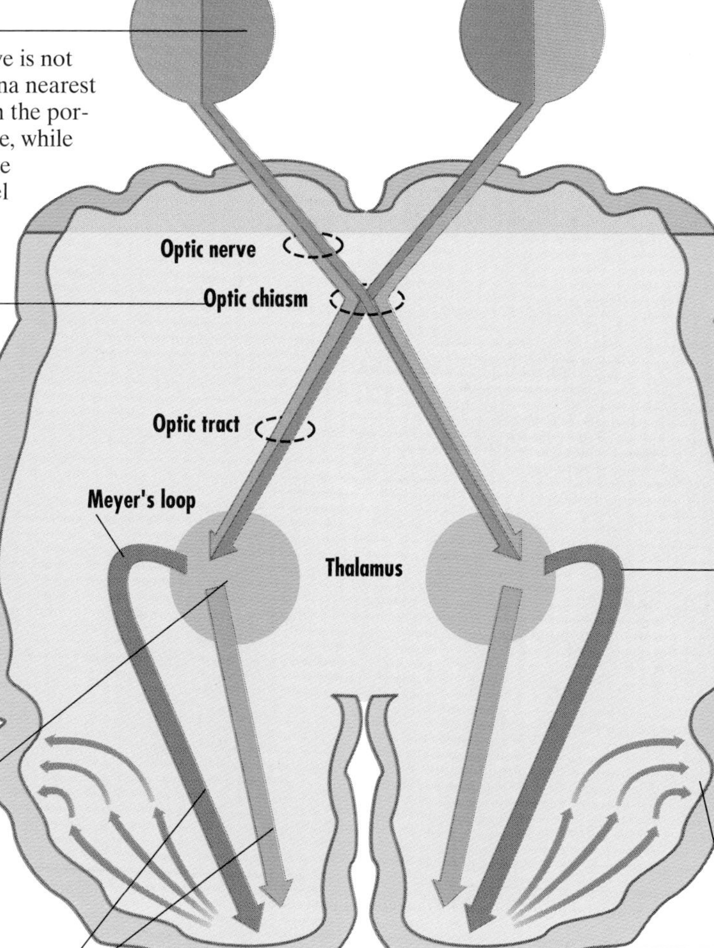

3 The *optic chiasm* (crossing) marks the end of the optic nerves and the beginning of the optic tracts. Here, the axons from the medial portion of each retina cross over to the opposite side of the brain, while the axons from the lateral portion of both retinas remain on their original side. So, while the optic nerves are made of axons from only one eye, the optic tracts are made of fibers from both eyes. (This difference between the optic nerves and the optic tracts helps in locating the cause of an eye problem. If vision is lost in only one eye, the problem is probably in the optic nerve or in the eye itself—anywhere before the optic chiasm.)

4 The nerve fibers of the optic tracts travel to the thalamus, where they synapse. From the thalamus, the visual pathways spread out along different courses to form the optic radiation.

5 The *optic radiation* is a group of nerve fibers that carries sight impulses from the thalamus to the primary visual cortex, which is found in the occipital lobe and is the most important reception area for sight in the brain. Colors of objects are probably first identified in the primary visual cortex.

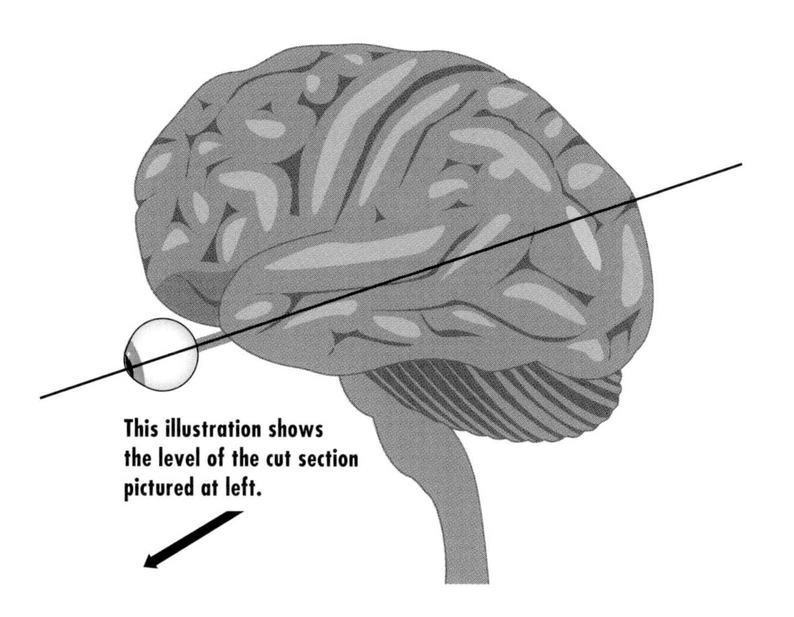

8 Our eyes gather more information than what is consciously "seen" by the cortex. Subconscious visual pathways regulate the pupil's response to light and also change the focus of the eyes for close or distant objects. Pathways from the eyes to the hypothalamus help to regulate the body's cyclic responses to day and night.

7 Some of the visual pathways loop into the temporal lobe before they continue onward to the occipital cortex. This diversion is called Meyer's loop. A stroke or tumor affecting the temporal lobe can interrupt Meyer's loop and can cause blindness in the upper portion of the field of vision.

6 From the primary visual cortex, impulses for sight pass to the *secondary visual cortex*, most of which lies in the occipital lobes, but some parts also spill over into nearby areas of the parietal and temporal lobes. In the secondary visual cortex, vision signals are analyzed for their finer points—surface textures, complex color shades, structural details, and three-dimensional position in space. Reading and the ability to recognize familiar objects are also located here.

Hearing: From the Ear to the Cortex

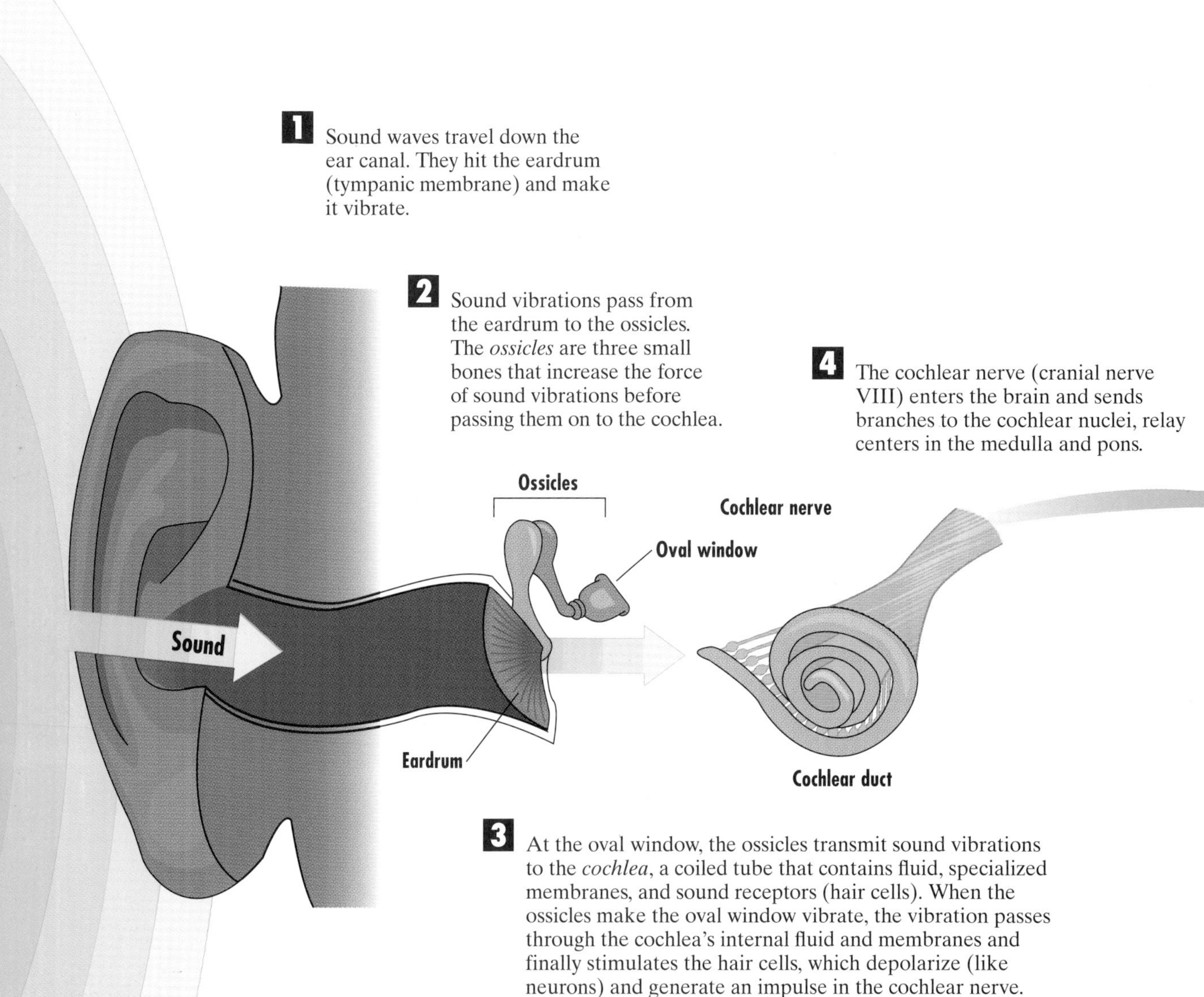

1 Sound waves travel down the ear canal. They hit the eardrum (tympanic membrane) and make it vibrate.

2 Sound vibrations pass from the eardrum to the ossicles. The *ossicles* are three small bones that increase the force of sound vibrations before passing them on to the cochlea.

3 At the oval window, the ossicles transmit sound vibrations to the *cochlea*, a coiled tube that contains fluid, specialized membranes, and sound receptors (hair cells). When the ossicles make the oval window vibrate, the vibration passes through the cochlea's internal fluid and membranes and finally stimulates the hair cells, which depolarize (like neurons) and generate an impulse in the cochlear nerve.

4 The cochlear nerve (cranial nerve VIII) enters the brain and sends branches to the cochlear nuclei, relay centers in the medulla and pons.

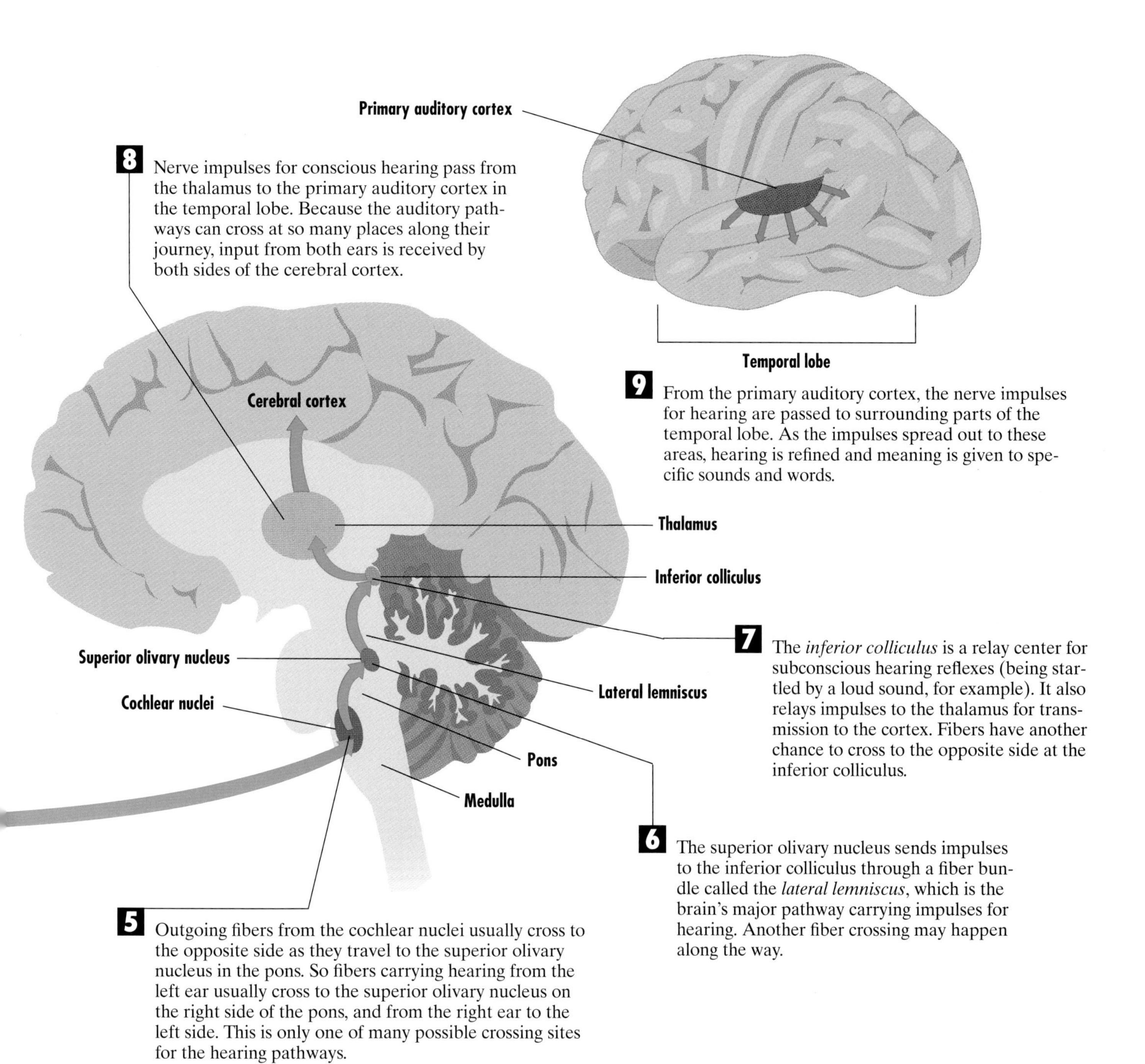

8 Nerve impulses for conscious hearing pass from the thalamus to the primary auditory cortex in the temporal lobe. Because the auditory pathways can cross at so many places along their journey, input from both ears is received by both sides of the cerebral cortex.

9 From the primary auditory cortex, the nerve impulses for hearing are passed to surrounding parts of the temporal lobe. As the impulses spread out to these areas, hearing is refined and meaning is given to specific sounds and words.

7 The *inferior colliculus* is a relay center for subconscious hearing reflexes (being startled by a loud sound, for example). It also relays impulses to the thalamus for transmission to the cortex. Fibers have another chance to cross to the opposite side at the inferior colliculus.

6 The superior olivary nucleus sends impulses to the inferior colliculus through a fiber bundle called the *lateral lemniscus*, which is the brain's major pathway carrying impulses for hearing. Another fiber crossing may happen along the way.

5 Outgoing fibers from the cochlear nuclei usually cross to the opposite side as they travel to the superior olivary nucleus in the pons. So fibers carrying hearing from the left ear usually cross to the superior olivary nucleus on the right side of the pons, and from the right ear to the left side. This is only one of many possible crossing sites for the hearing pathways.

WORLDWIDE ALERT Besides the pathway shown here, the brain has important neural side roads that are activated by sudden loud noises. These pathways alert the cerebellum and many other parts of the brain to be ready to respond to danger.

Speech: Anatomy and Physiology of a Miracle

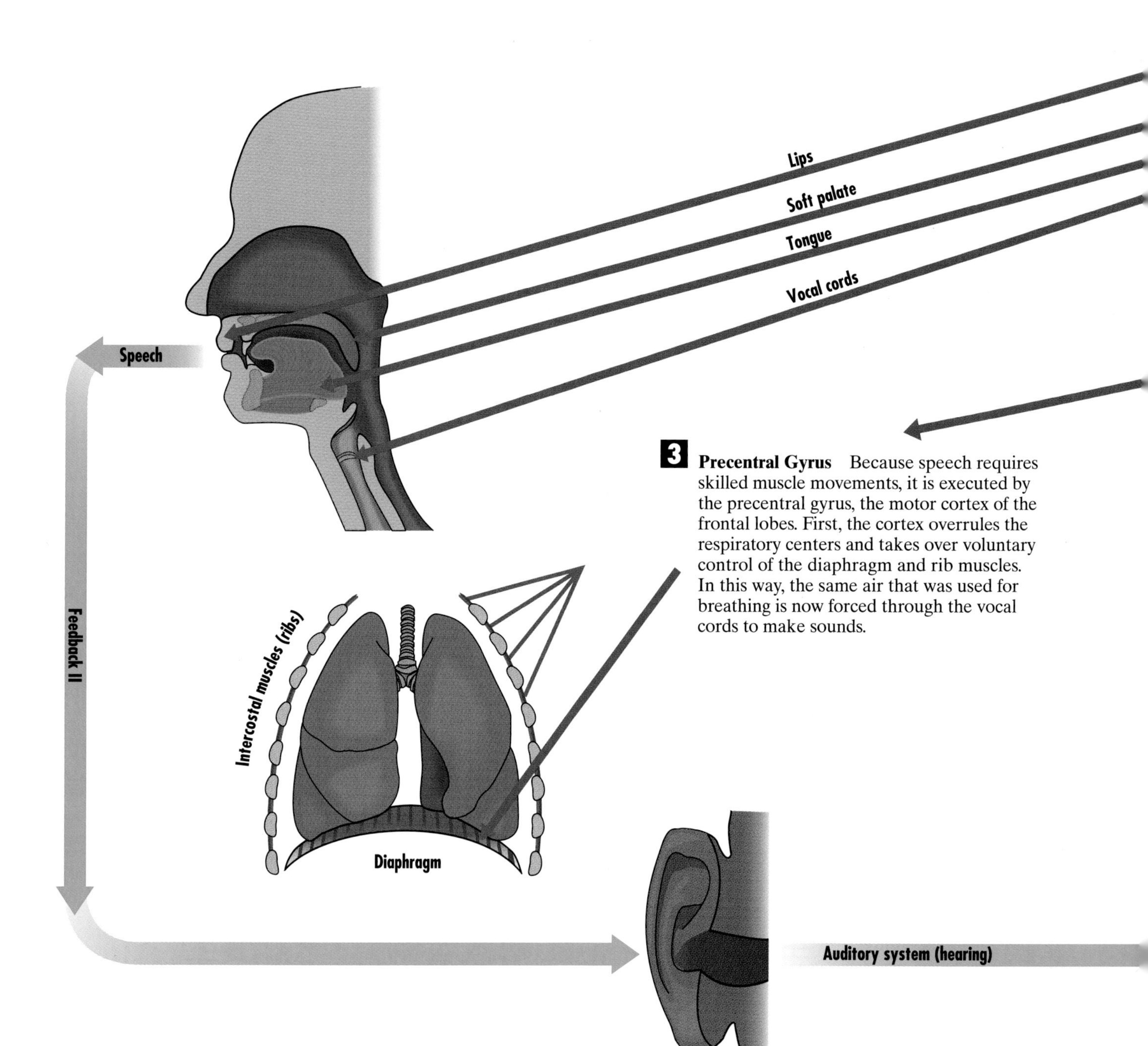

3 Precentral Gyrus Because speech requires skilled muscle movements, it is executed by the precentral gyrus, the motor cortex of the frontal lobes. First, the cortex overrules the respiratory centers and takes over voluntary control of the diaphragm and rib muscles. In this way, the same air that was used for breathing is now forced through the vocal cords to make sounds.

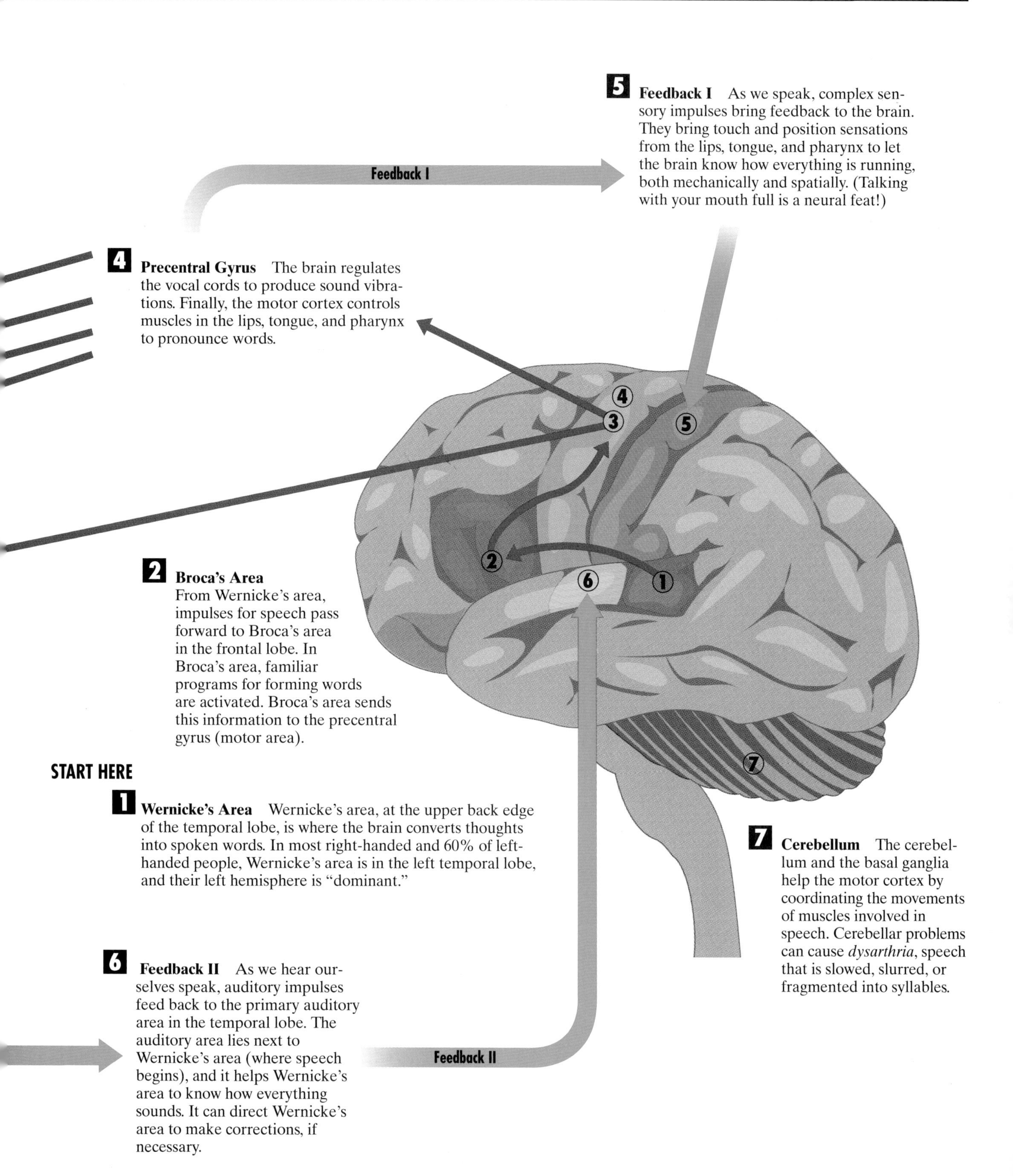

5 Feedback I As we speak, complex sensory impulses bring feedback to the brain. They bring touch and position sensations from the lips, tongue, and pharynx to let the brain know how everything is running, both mechanically and spatially. (Talking with your mouth full is a neural feat!)

4 Precentral Gyrus The brain regulates the vocal cords to produce sound vibrations. Finally, the motor cortex controls muscles in the lips, tongue, and pharynx to pronounce words.

2 Broca's Area
From Wernicke's area, impulses for speech pass forward to Broca's area in the frontal lobe. In Broca's area, familiar programs for forming words are activated. Broca's area sends this information to the precentral gyrus (motor area).

START HERE

1 Wernicke's Area Wernicke's area, at the upper back edge of the temporal lobe, is where the brain converts thoughts into spoken words. In most right-handed and 60% of left-handed people, Wernicke's area is in the left temporal lobe, and their left hemisphere is "dominant."

7 Cerebellum The cerebellum and the basal ganglia help the motor cortex by coordinating the movements of muscles involved in speech. Cerebellar problems can cause *dysarthria*, speech that is slowed, slurred, or fragmented into syllables.

6 Feedback II As we hear ourselves speak, auditory impulses feed back to the primary auditory area in the temporal lobe. The auditory area lies next to Wernicke's area (where speech begins), and it helps Wernicke's area to know how everything sounds. It can direct Wernicke's area to make corrections, if necessary.

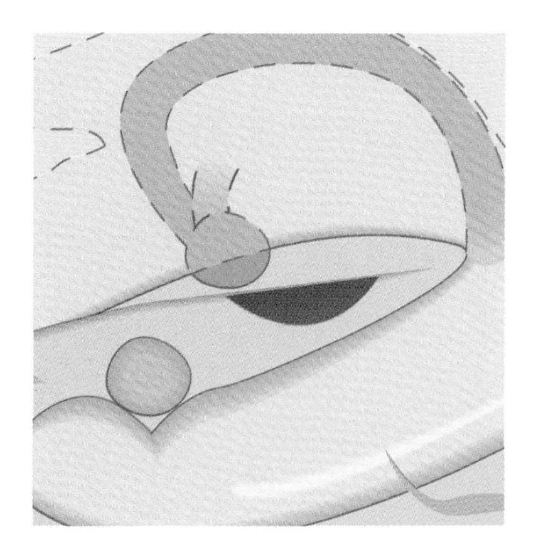

The Brain and Emotion
Passionate Circuits

PASSION AND EMOTION are part of the spark of life. They color the brain's sensory input and drive its motor responses. They give the brain its motivation and provide the psychic energy behind the intellect's power to create and destroy. Like the human world, the neural world is challenged to direct its passions into channels that are self-preserving. The brain does this through the limbic system.

The *limbic system* is an odd group of connected structures that encircles the central core of the brain. Part of the limbic system lies near the corpus callosum, part extends into the frontal and temporal lobes, and part descends into the hypothalamus. The limbic system also includes parts of the cerebral cortex, as well as the the amygdala (one of the basal ganglia). Stimulation of various limbic structures can cause rage, fear, aggression, or feelings linked to sexuality. These emotions are channeled through limbic circuits to arrive at the hypothalamus, where they have the potential to trigger dramatic changes in the functions of vital organs. Although scientific exploration of the limbic system is only beginning, four of its structures are especially intriguing: the hippocampus, the amygdala, the cingulate gyrus, and the hypothalamus.

The *hippocampus* is found deep in the temporal lobes, in a part of the brain that is very primitive and old in evolutionary terms. The hippocampus probably plays a role in learning, since it seems to help the brain decide which information will be stored as memories. The *amygdala* lies near the hippocampus, and it receives extensive input from the cortical areas for hearing and vision. The amygdala is linked to feelings of rage and fear and may help the brain decide what type of behavior is appropriate for a particular situation. The *cingulate gyrus* lies directly above the corpus callosum, which is the major bridge of white matter between the hemispheres. The strategic position of the cingulate gyrus may allow it to act as a link between the important sensory and motor areas of the cortex and the emotional circuits of the limbic system. The cingulate gyrus may be a mediator between the "higher" neural regions (the cerebral hemispheres) and the more primitive, passionate core of the brain.

The *hypothalamus* receives input from all parts of the limbic system and exerts its control over the body's appetites, hormones and vital functions. The hypothalamus and all its fascinating relationships are worthy of a separate chapter—the next stop on our neural exploration.

The Neural World's Emotional Core: The Limbic System

1 Corpus Callosum The corpus callosum is the great bridge of white matter that connects the left and right sides of the brain. It is not part of the limbic system, but it is a good landmark for locating parts of the limbic system.

2 Cingulate Gyrus The cingulate gyrus is the ridge of cerebral cortex that lies directly above the corpus callosum on both sides of the brain. As part of the limbic system, the cingulate gyrus mediates between the intellectual cortex and the emotional limbic system.

3 Mammillary Bodies The mammillary bodies (left and right) are two swellings near the hypothalamus that are part of the limbic system. They are involved in controlling primitive reflexes of the tongue and throat muscles used in eating.

4 Olfactory Bulb The olfactory bulb is part of the olfactory nerve (sense of smell) and also part of the limbic system. It brings input from the sense of smell to the frontal and temporal lobes of the cerebral cortex and to the hypothalamus. It provides a very direct route to link smell with emotion, which may explain why we find perfumes so exciting.

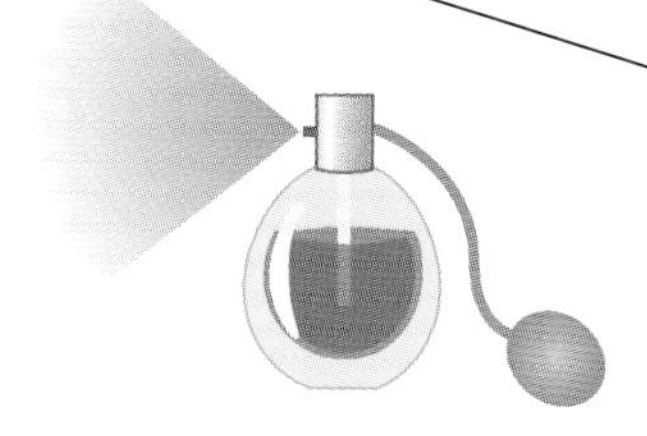

5 Amygdala The amygdala, a complex of nuclei (specialized groups of neuron cell bodies), may be the limbic system's major receiving area for all types of sensory information, with especially strong input from visual and auditory areas. Stimulating the amygdala can cause rage, fear, and sexual feelings and can signal the hypothalamus to affect heart function, blood pressure, digestion, and hormone secretion. The amygdala may also be the neural area that determines which behavior is appropriate for a particular situation.

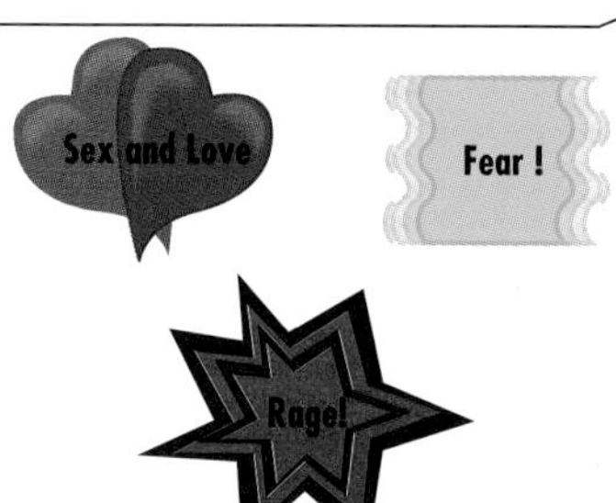

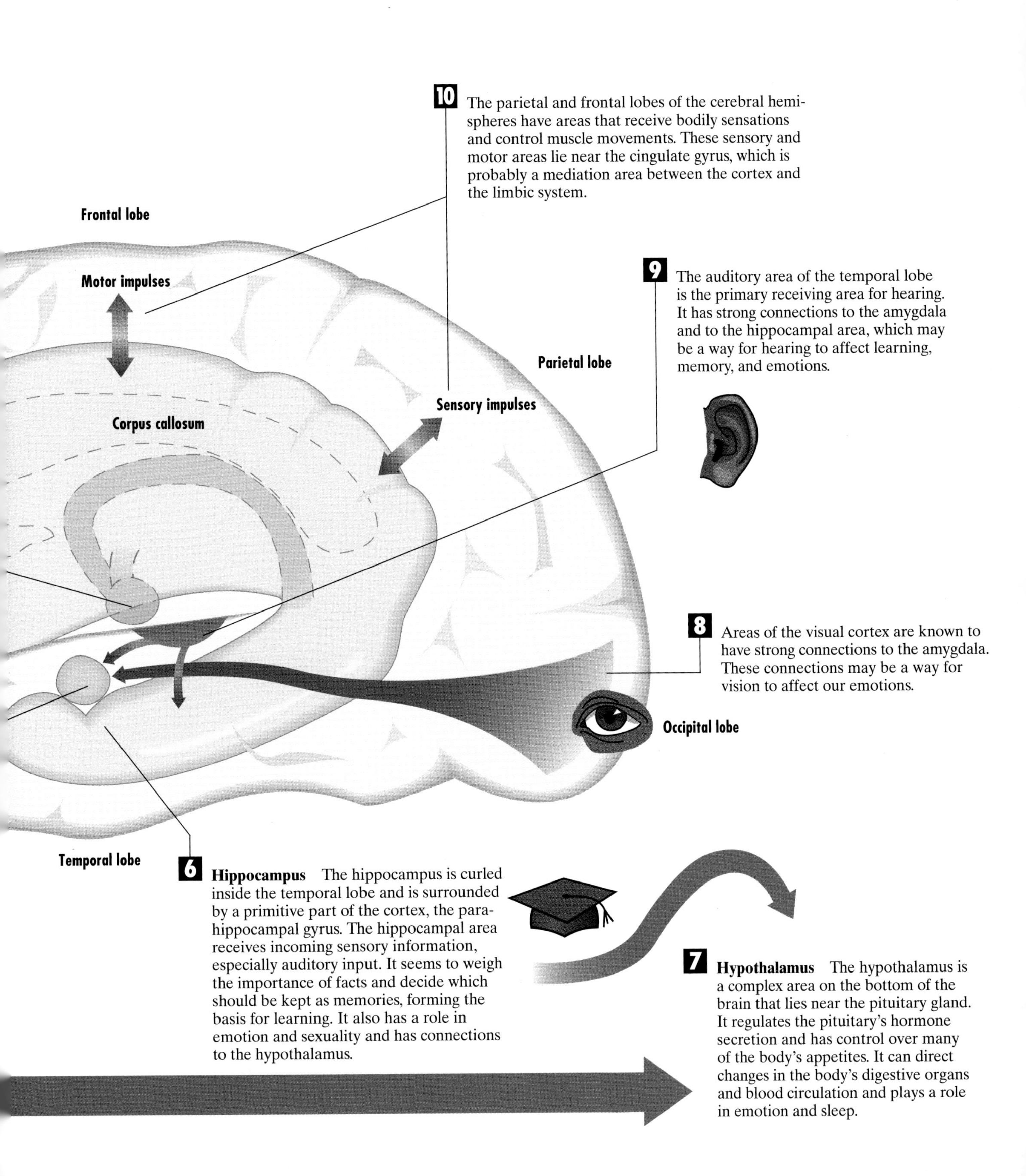

10 The parietal and frontal lobes of the cerebral hemispheres have areas that receive bodily sensations and control muscle movements. These sensory and motor areas lie near the cingulate gyrus, which is probably a mediation area between the cortex and the limbic system.

9 The auditory area of the temporal lobe is the primary receiving area for hearing. It has strong connections to the amygdala and to the hippocampal area, which may be a way for hearing to affect learning, memory, and emotions.

8 Areas of the visual cortex are known to have strong connections to the amygdala. These connections may be a way for vision to affect our emotions.

6 **Hippocampus** The hippocampus is curled inside the temporal lobe and is surrounded by a primitive part of the cortex, the parahippocampal gyrus. The hippocampal area receives incoming sensory information, especially auditory input. It seems to weigh the importance of facts and decide which should be kept as memories, forming the basis for learning. It also has a role in emotion and sexuality and has connections to the hypothalamus.

7 **Hypothalamus** The hypothalamus is a complex area on the bottom of the brain that lies near the pituitary gland. It regulates the pituitary's hormone secretion and has control over many of the body's appetites. It can direct changes in the body's digestive organs and blood circulation and plays a role in emotion and sleep.

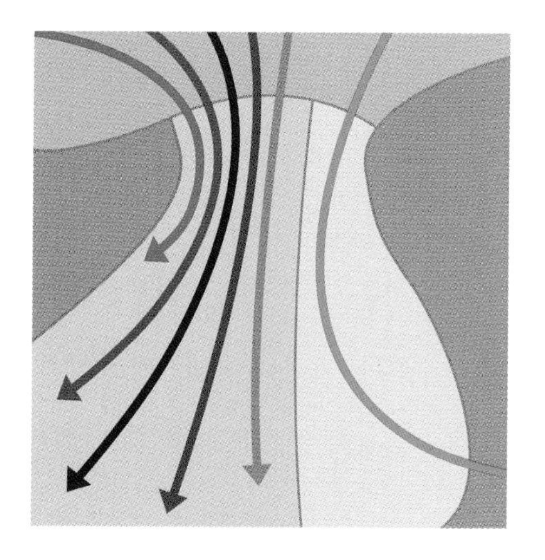

The Hypothalamus
Climate Control and More

THE SLINGS AND ARROWS of outrageous fortune are everywhere in the human world, and human beings are always confronting forces beyond their control. In the brain, life is much more predictable and regulated, because the brain has something that the human world does not: the hypothalamus.

The hypothalamus has it all covered. It regulates the body's internal climate, temperature, water economy, and energy resources. The hypothalamus triggers sweating when the body is hot and shivering when the body is cold. It creates thirst when the internal climate is dry and increases urine formation when there is fluid overload. It regulates the body's food intake, governing both hunger and satiety. And it influences the heart rate and blood pressure.

As a major outlet for the limbic system, the hypothalamus also affects the body's emotional climate. There are hypothalamic areas that play a role in our feelings of rage and tranquility, fighting and fear. The hypothalamus can awaken the body's strongest appetites, engaging our human drives for sex and for food.

Since the hypothalamus lies directly above the pituitary gland, it takes the liberty of regulating the pituitary as well. The hypothalamus produces a series of *releasing hormones* and *inhibiting hormones* that tell the pituitary when to begin and when to end its hormone production. By regulating the pituitary's hormones, the hypothalamus can oversee the body's growth, its puberty and reproductive capabilities, its metabolism, and its hormonal response to trauma and stress. Through subconscious input from the eyes, the hypothalamus can also act as an internal timekeeper, linking the cyclic release of some pituitary hormones to the passage of hours or days.

Our arrival at the hypothalamus marks the end of our basic tour of the brain. As we recall our journey, it is possible to make creative speculations about the places we've visited. We can trace prospective routes that begin in a cranial nerve, pass to the cortex, enter the limbic system, jump down to the hypothalamus, and finally end in secretion of pituitary hormones. There is so much of the brain left to discover. A route that we propose today may be mapped by a neural scientist tomorrow.

The brain is a mysterious world of elegant interweavings. The more we explore it, the more we appreciate how wonderfully and beautifully it is designed.

The Hypothalamus: Location and Anatomy

1 Using the corpus callosum as a landmark, we can visualize the location of some of the hypothalamus's major incoming tracts. Also, notice the physical connection between the hypothalamus and the pituitary gland.

2 Tracts of white matter curve below the corpus callosum. They help connect the limbic system's amygdala and hippocampus to the hypothalamus.

3 A series of tracts that begin in the frontal lobe's olfactory areas (responsible for sense of smell) brings incoming information to the hypothalamus. These connections may allow environmental smells to influence our emotional drives.

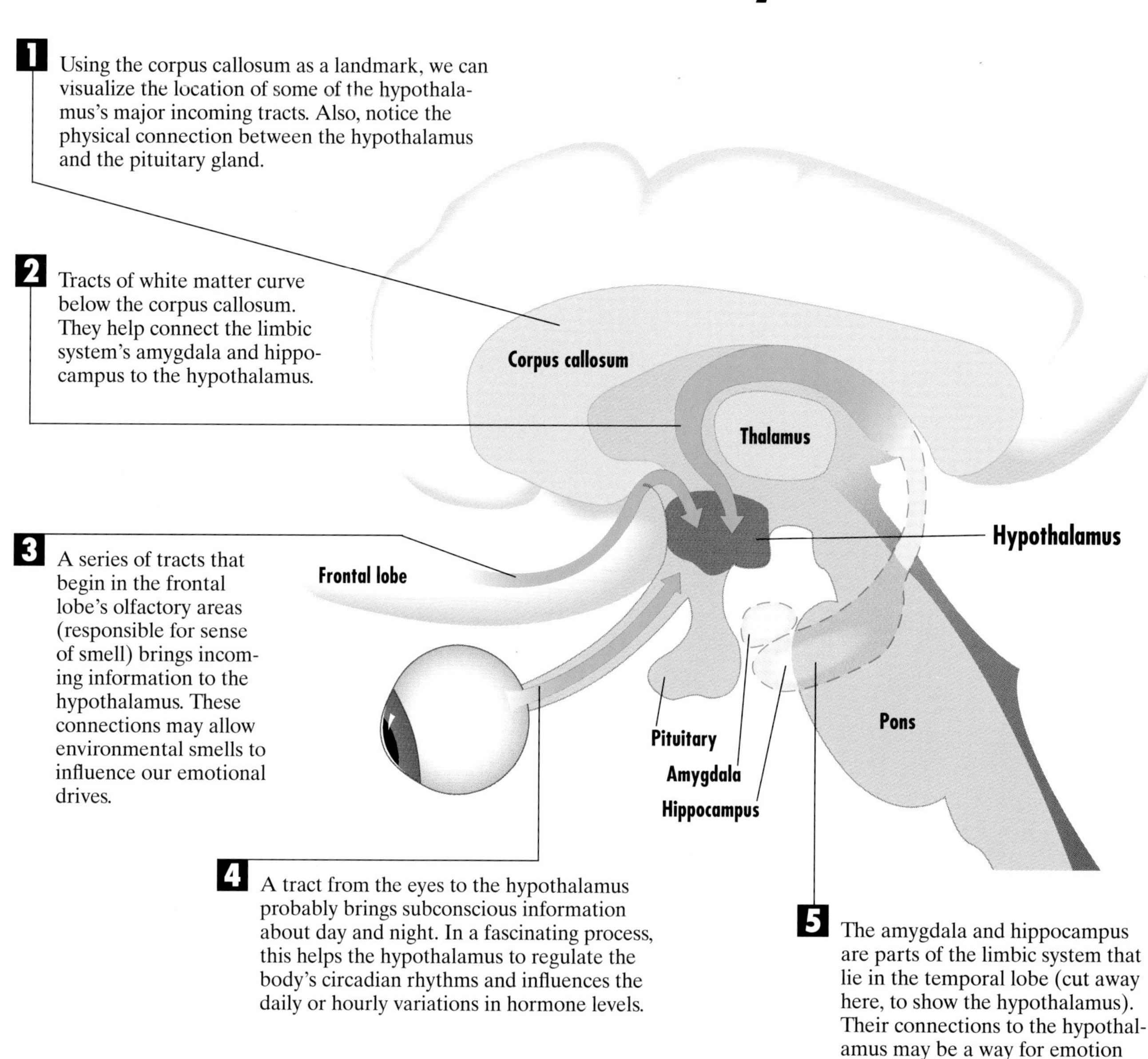

4 A tract from the eyes to the hypothalamus probably brings subconscious information about day and night. In a fascinating process, this helps the hypothalamus to regulate the body's circadian rhythms and influences the daily or hourly variations in hormone levels.

5 The amygdala and hippocampus are parts of the limbic system that lie in the temporal lobe (cut away here, to show the hypothalamus). Their connections to the hypothalamus may be a way for emotion and memory to influence the actions of the hypothalamus.

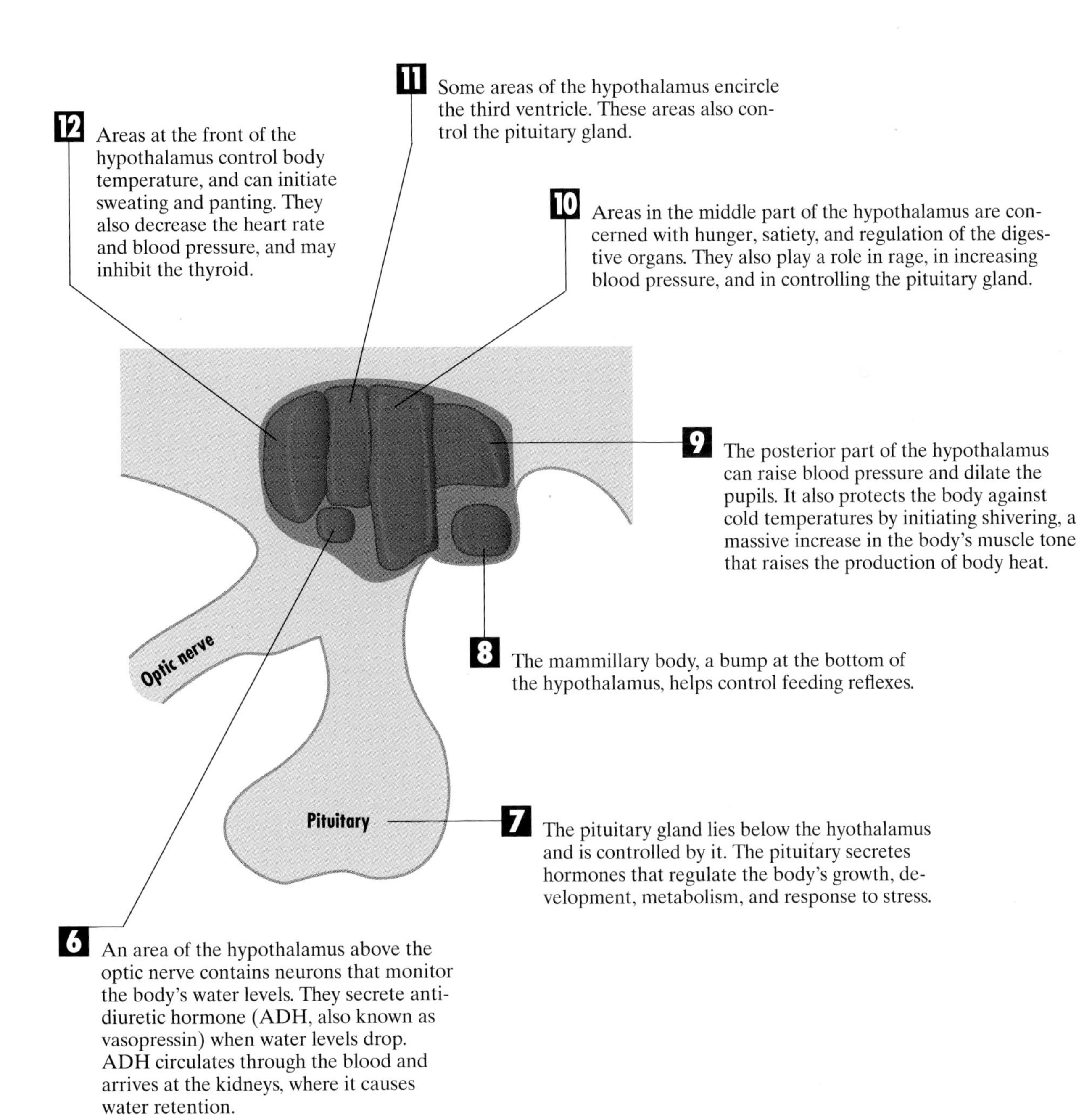
6 An area of the hypothalamus above the optic nerve contains neurons that monitor the body's water levels. They secrete anti-diuretic hormone (ADH, also known as vasopressin) when water levels drop. ADH circulates through the blood and arrives at the kidneys, where it causes water retention.
7 The pituitary gland lies below the hyothalamus and is controlled by it. The pituitary secretes hormones that regulate the body's growth, development, metabolism, and response to stress.
8 The mammillary body, a bump at the bottom of the hypothalamus, helps control feeding reflexes.
9 The posterior part of the hypothalamus can raise blood pressure and dilate the pupils. It also protects the body against cold temperatures by initiating shivering, a massive increase in the body's muscle tone that raises the production of body heat.
10 Areas in the middle part of the hypothalamus are concerned with hunger, satiety, and regulation of the digestive organs. They also play a role in rage, in increasing blood pressure, and in controlling the pituitary gland.
11 Some areas of the hypothalamus encircle the third ventricle. These areas also control the pituitary gland.
12 Areas at the front of the hypothalamus control body temperature, and can initiate sweating and panting. They also decrease the heart rate and blood pressure, and may inhibit the thyroid.
Optic nerve
Pituitary

Hypothalamic Messengers: Neural Control of the Pituitary

1 Neurons in specialized areas of the hypothalamus secrete chemical messengers called releasing hormones and inhibiting hormones. These messengers enter the circulation between the hypothalamus and the pituitary. They are carried by the blood to the anterior (front) part of the pituitary gland, where they affect secretion of pituitary hormones. Releasing hormones from the hypothalamus cause the pituitary to release, or secrete, its hormones while inhibiting hormones inhibit, or block, that secretion.

2 The hypothalamus has both a releasing hormone and an inhibiting hormone to regulate the pituitary's secretion of growth hormone. Growth hormone directs the body's cells to make more protein, and it helps the body grow.

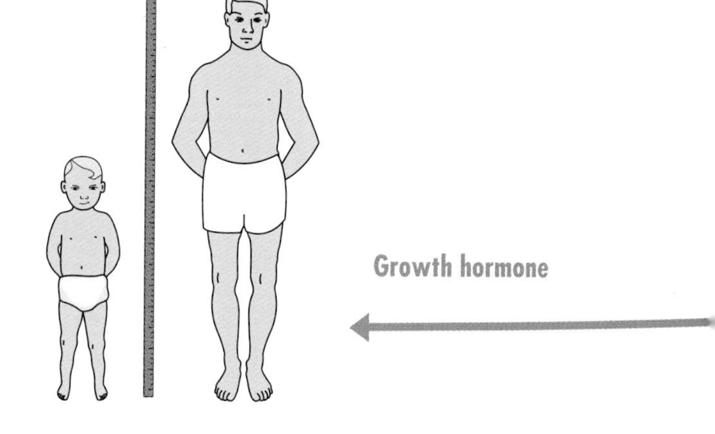

3 The hypothalamus has a releasing hormone that makes the pituitary secrete ACTH (adrenocorticotropin). ACTH makes the adrenal glands secrete cortisol in response to stresses like trauma or infection. Cortisol helps the body mobilize its energy resources, like carbohydrates (sugars) and fats, and can help prevent inflammation.

Infection
Trauma
Stress
Glucose
ACTH
Cortisol

4 The hypothalamus has a releasing hormone that regulates the pituitary's production of FSH and LH. FSH and LH circulate to the sex organs to direct production of sex hormones, which are important in reproduction, in maintaining the body's sex organs and secondary sexual characteristics (pubic hair, beard, breasts), and in regulating women's menstrual cycles.

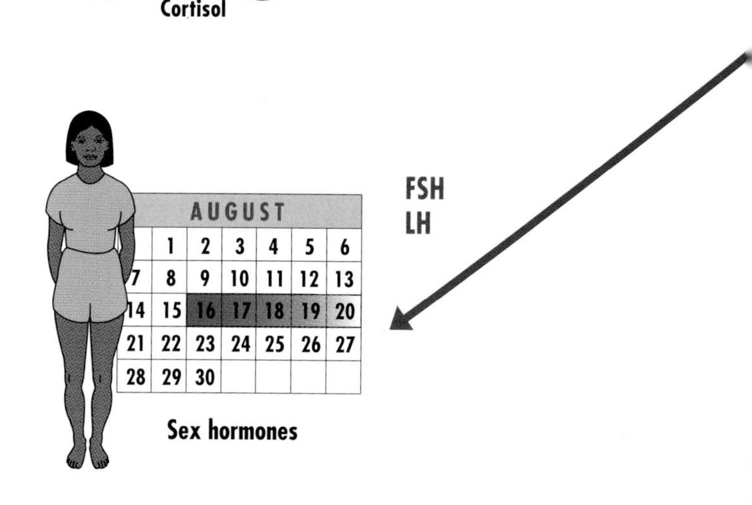

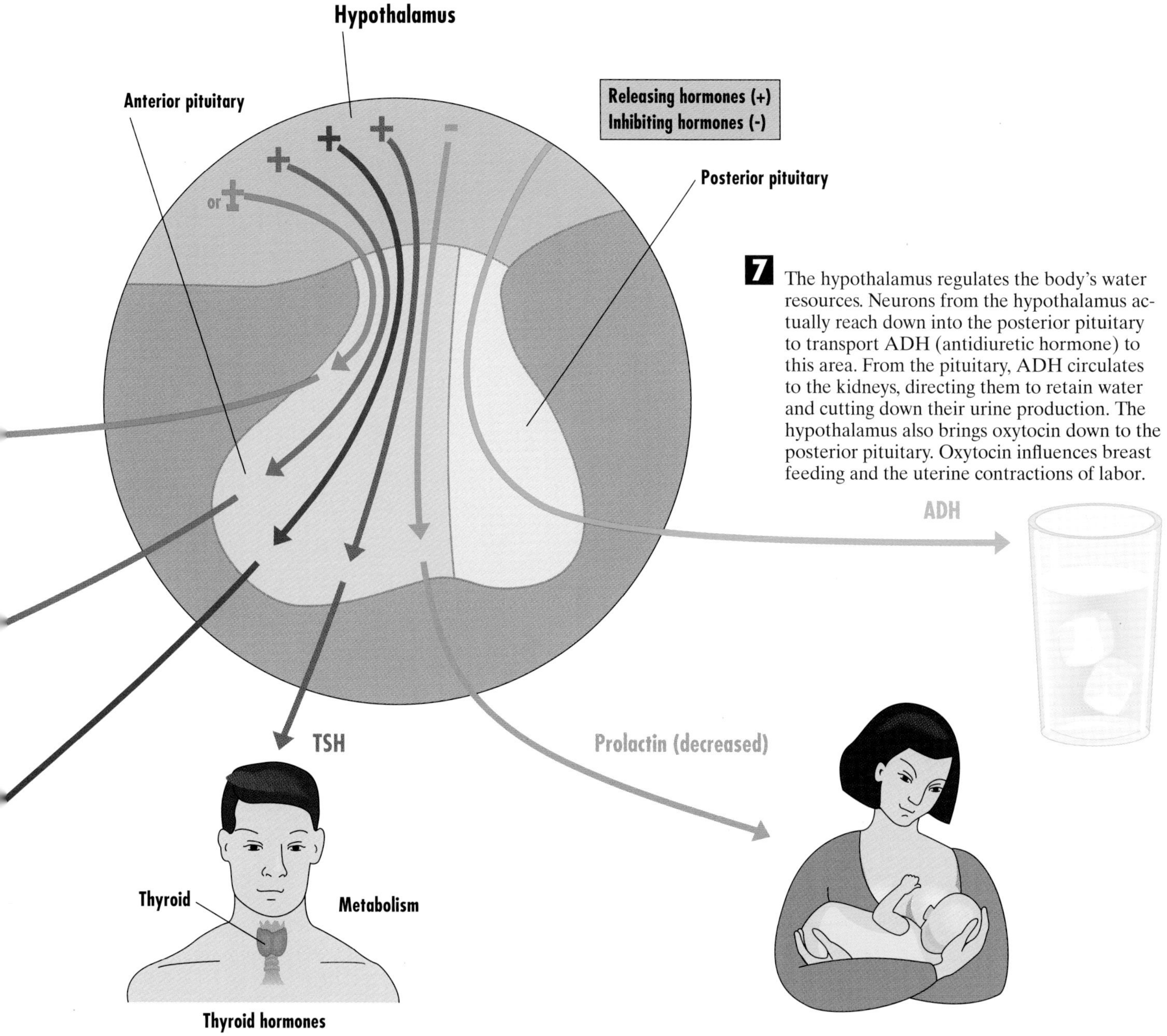

Hypothalamus

Anterior pituitary

Releasing hormones (+)
Inhibiting hormones (-)

Posterior pituitary

or

7 The hypothalamus regulates the body's water resources. Neurons from the hypothalamus actually reach down into the posterior pituitary to transport ADH (antidiuretic hormone) to this area. From the pituitary, ADH circulates to the kidneys, directing them to retain water and cutting down their urine production. The hypothalamus also brings oxytocin down to the posterior pituitary. Oxytocin influences breast feeding and the uterine contractions of labor.

ADH

TSH

Prolactin (decreased)

Thyroid

Metabolism

Thyroid hormones

5 The hypothalamus secretes a releasing hormone that makes the pituitary produce TSH. TSH (thyroid-stimulating hormone) stimulates the thyroid to produce its own thyroid hormones, which regulate the body's metabolism.

6 The hypothalamus has an inhibiting factor that cuts the pituitary's production of prolactin. Prolactin controls the production of breast milk.

From Famine to Feast: The Hypothalamus and Hunger

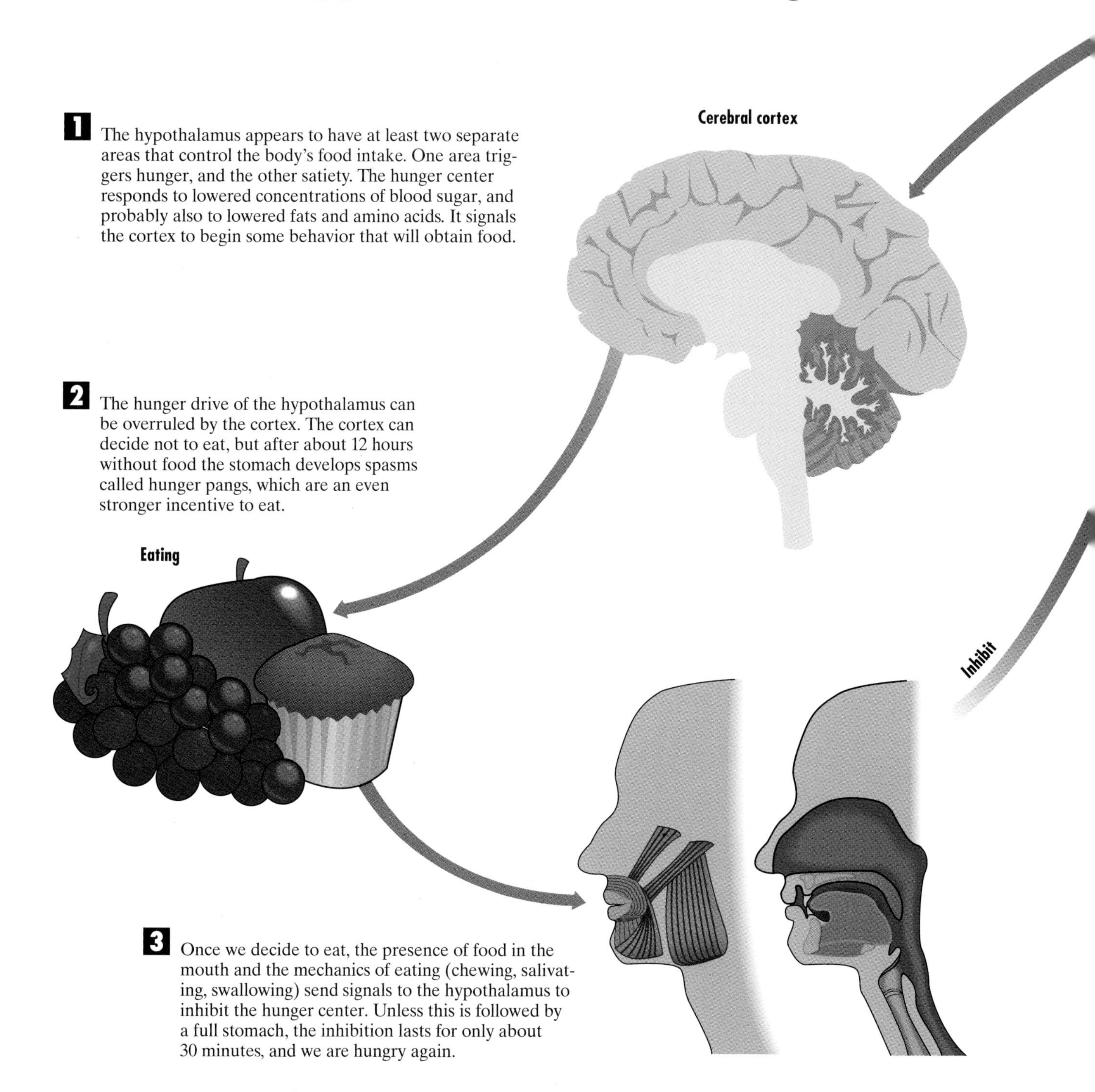

1 The hypothalamus appears to have at least two separate areas that control the body's food intake. One area triggers hunger, and the other satiety. The hunger center responds to lowered concentrations of blood sugar, and probably also to lowered fats and amino acids. It signals the cortex to begin some behavior that will obtain food.

2 The hunger drive of the hypothalamus can be overruled by the cortex. The cortex can decide not to eat, but after about 12 hours without food the stomach develops spasms called hunger pangs, which are an even stronger incentive to eat.

3 Once we decide to eat, the presence of food in the mouth and the mechanics of eating (chewing, salivating, swallowing) send signals to the hypothalamus to inhibit the hunger center. Unless this is followed by a full stomach, the inhibition lasts for only about 30 minutes, and we are hungry again.

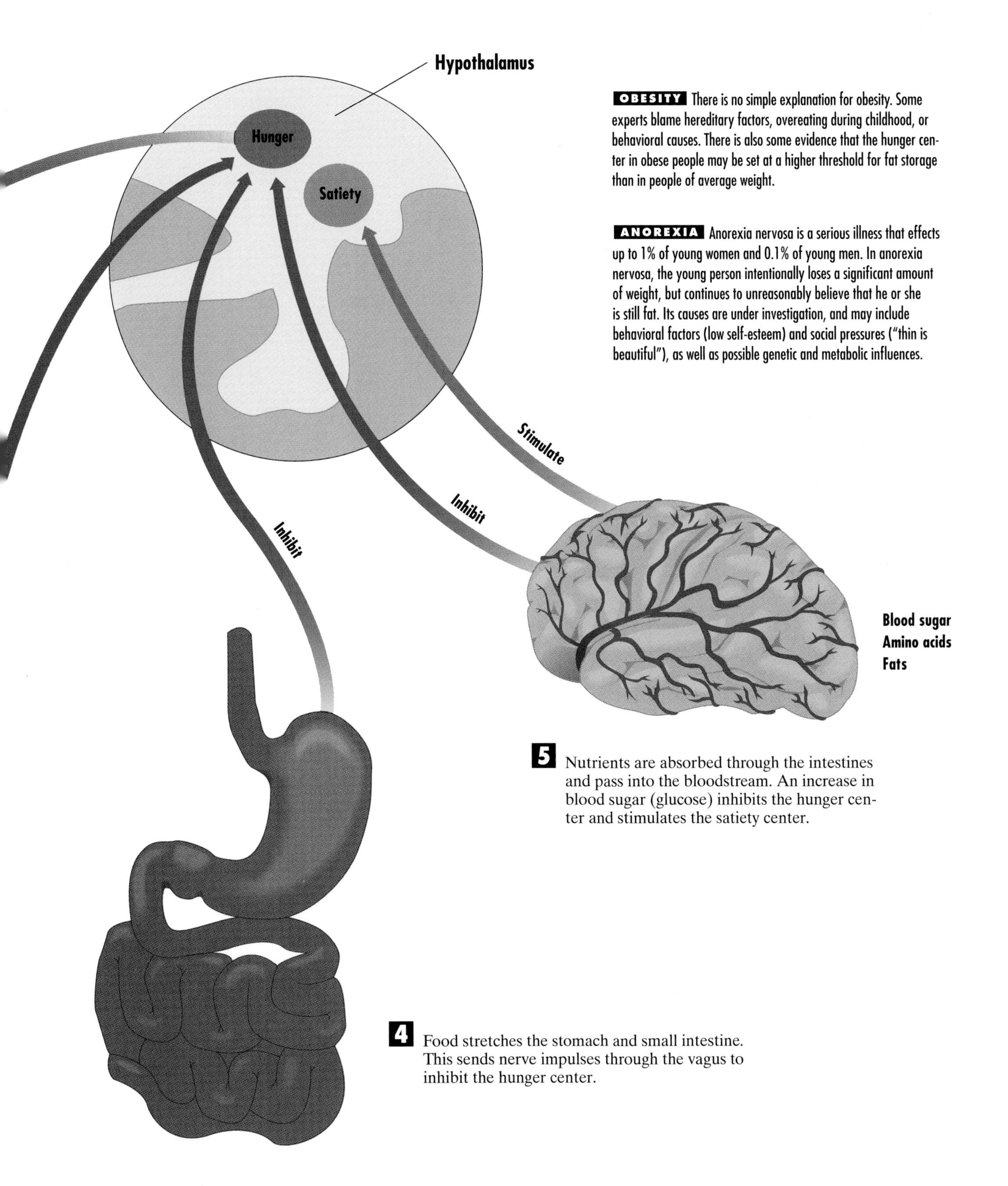

OBESITY There is no simple explanation for obesity. Some experts blame hereditary factors, overeating during childhood, or behavioral causes. There is also some evidence that the hunger center in obese people may be set at a higher threshold for fat storage than in people of average weight.

ANOREXIA Anorexia nervosa is a serious illness that effects up to 1% of young women and 0.1% of young men. In anorexia nervosa, the young person intentionally loses a significant amount of weight, but continues to unreasonably believe that he or she is still fat. Its causes are under investigation, and may include behavioral factors (low self-esteem) and social pressures ("thin is beautiful"), as well as possible genetic and metabolic influences.

5 Nutrients are absorbed through the intestines and pass into the bloodstream. An increase in blood sugar (glucose) inhibits the hunger center and stimulates the satiety center.

4 Food stretches the stomach and small intestine. This sends nerve impulses through the vagus to inhibit the hunger center.

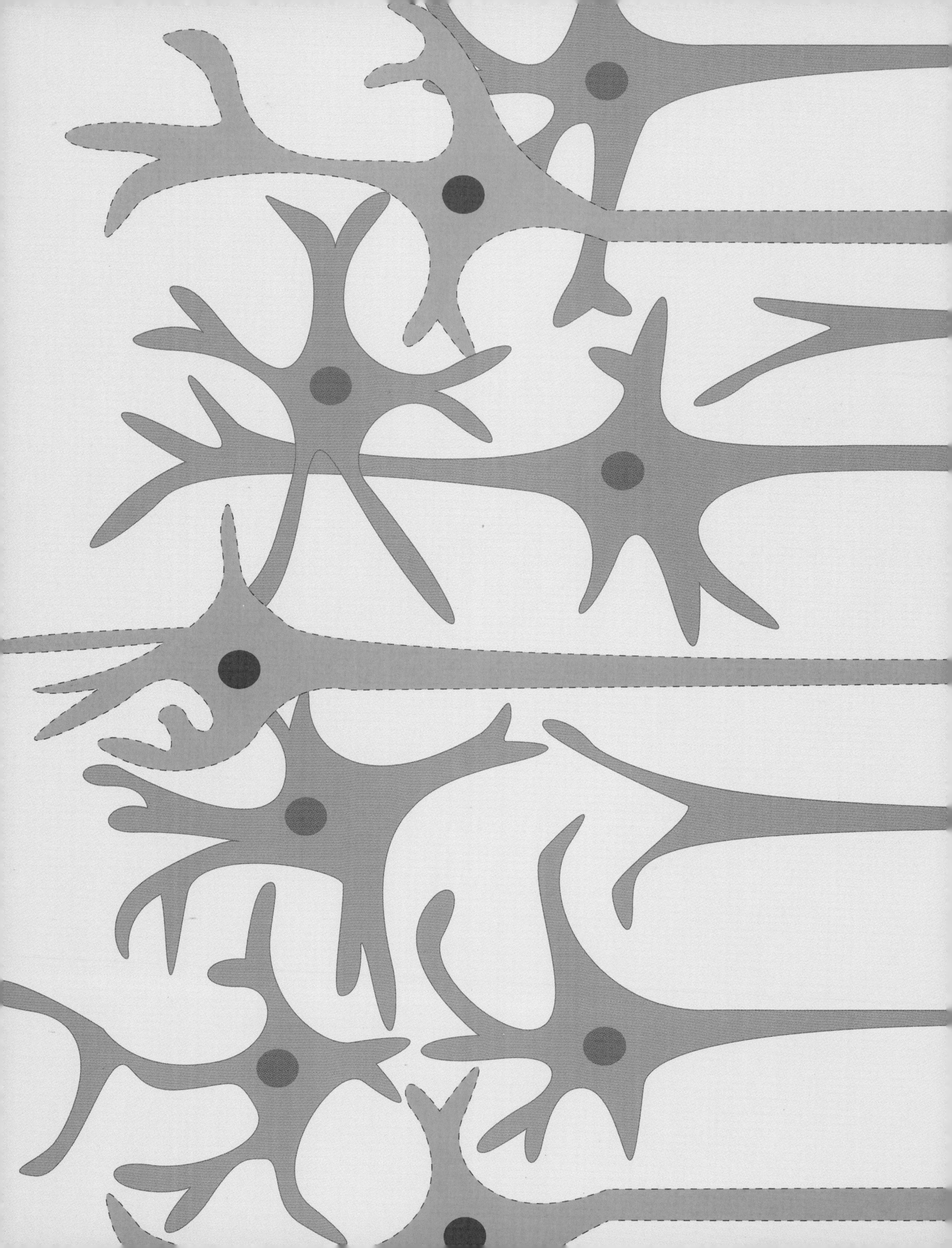

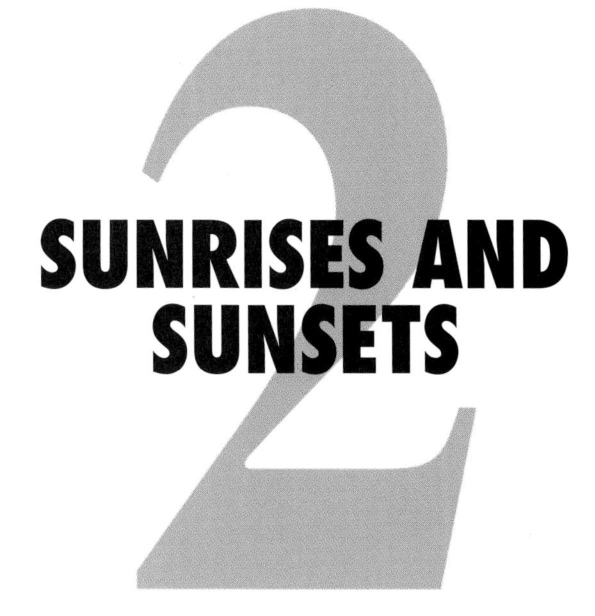

SUNRISES AND SUNSETS

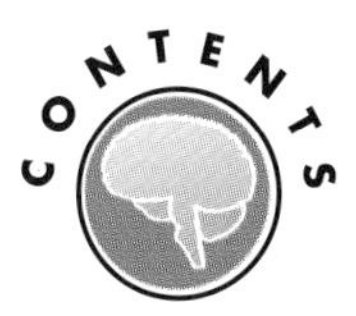

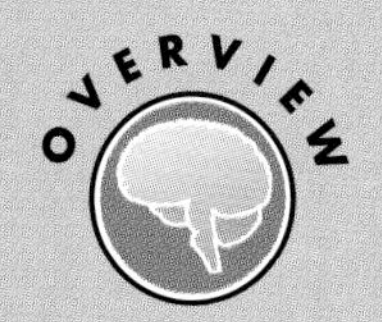
OVERVIEW

SOME PEOPLE BELIEVE that fate is the sum of substance and environmental history, that worlds live and die depending on what they are made of and what outside influences affect them over time. The brain, like any planet, has both substance and history. Together, they affect the brain's quality of life and ultimately affect its death as well.

As we have already seen, the substance of the human brain is made of living cells. So, unlike our planet Earth, the brain does not have a separate geology and biology—its substance and its population are one and the same.

Before birth, the structure of the brain is outlined and constructed according to hereditary factors found in the genetic blueprint of DNA. What begins as a simple tube of embryonic tissue develops over nine months into a complex system of intellect, reflexes, and emotions. The neuron population that arises before birth comprises all the neurons that the brain will ever have. Any environmental misfortune that affects the neurons, especially in the first six months of fetal life, may be reflected in the structure of the brain for a lifetime.

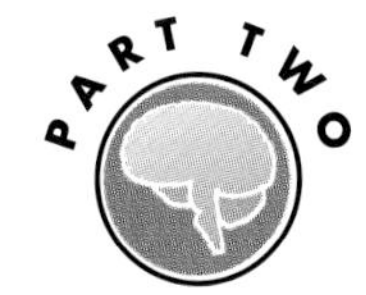

Likewise, after birth, the fate of the brain is linked to its environment. Good nutrition, together with a learning environment that is rich in sensory stimulation, can help neurons to grow bigger and to increase the complexity of their synapses. Neurons that are stimulated over and over again will experience measurable structural changes that form the basis for learning.

However, ultimately, the brain is a finite world. Perhaps more than any other organ, the brain begins to die as soon as it is born. A normal lifetime of wear may cause the loss of a million or more neurons daily, and these are not replaced. Add to this the extraordinary neuron losses that accompany a lifetime of small head traumas, illnesses of all kinds, and environmental toxins, and you see that the brain's survival is filled with daily risks. For a healthy brain to endure to old age, it must learn to recognize—and anticipate—danger. And it must learn to manipulate its environment, including everything from nutrition to emotional stress, for its own survival.

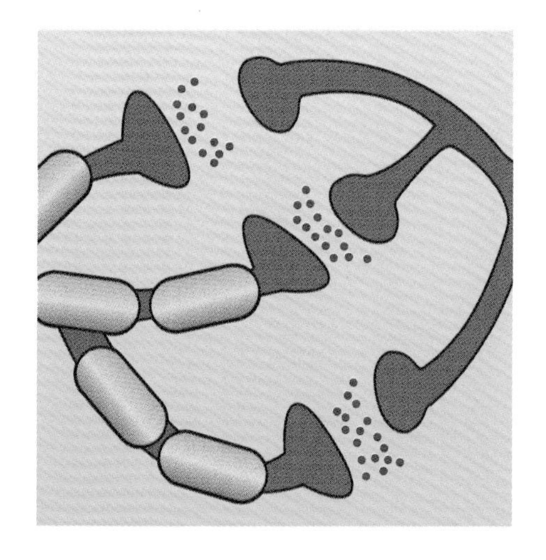

The Brain Grows and Learns
Sunrises

THE ORGANIZATION OF the human body gives primacy to the brain, and the brain controls other body organs for its own purposes. So, we might expect that the brain would develop early in the human embryo, and it does.

The brain begins as a tube of primitive neural tissue that forms on the twenty-third day of embryonic life, very early in the first trimester of pregnancy. Within another week, when the embryo is one month old, the cerebral hemispheres begin to form, and the heart beats. Neurons appear at about day 40, and reach their final population of billions by the time the embryo is only four months old. Primitive reflexes are present at three months and the outline of the corpus callosum is begun. Also at three months, respiratory movements appear, but only briefly (since the embryo is surrounded by fluid); they'll reappear at a more appropriate time (birth). By the time the fetus is about seven months old, neural control of digestive organs allows them to function as well as those of a newborn.

At birth, the brain sees its sunrise. All its neurons are in place, and it has already achieved about 30% of its adult size. Within the next two years of childhood, brain size will almost triple. White myelin, which is rare at birth, will be deposited around the axon fibers that form the brain's maturing white matter tracts. Growth, especially in the primary sensory, motor, and visual areas, will be remarkable.

As the brain grows, it learns. It establishes patterns of synapses between specific sequences of neurons, and it can recall these patterns at will. Neurons that are involved in the learned patterns actually undergo physical changes that make synaptic transmission easier. The exact nature of these physical changes is being studied. It may be that the neurons grow more axons or dendrites, that they make more neurotransmitter molecules, or that they can release these molecules over a greater area. There is still much to learn about learning.

For example, there is evidence that, in early childhood, frequently fired neurons may grow stronger and larger, while their unused neighbors just disappear. In this way, the brain's own electrical activity seems to sculpt the structure of its neuron populations for a lifetime. This sculpting may help the brain to structurally fit the stimulation it gets from its particular environment. But the neurons that disappear are gone forever.

The mechanisms for learning and memory are difficult to study in living human beings. Much of our information about the microscopic changes involved in learning comes from animal studies, particularly studies of very small animals with very simple nervous systems, like snails. Important information in humans often comes from people who have suffered a neural tragedy that has affected their memory systems. The location of their neural problem is correlated with its resulting memory deficit by using a kind of neurological detective work. This gives us clues about the way the brain learns.

For example, studies of amnesia victims have led scientists to believe that the brain must "rehearse" new information over and over again for 10 to 60 minutes before it can permanently remember it. Evidence for this comes from examining the time of onset of amnesia in people who have had either a concussion or general anesthesia immediately after learning something new.

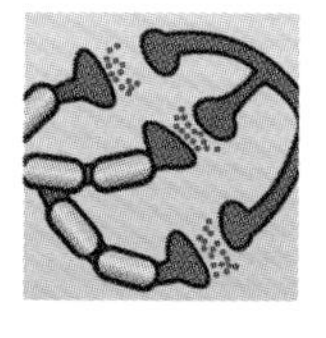

Also, scientists have found that people who have had their hippocampi surgically removed (a treatment for epilepsy) often cannot *form* new long-term memories after surgery, while people with problems in the thalamus may have trouble *retrieving* memories that have already been stored.

More and more, the evidence points to areas of the temporal lobe, especially the hippocampi and Wernicke's areas, as key control areas for learning and memory. Yet the exact storage areas for memories are not known, and even people with massive destruction of both cerebral hemispheres have been able to retain some of their strongest and dearest long-term memories.

No discussion of the growing brain would be complete without mentioning the problems that arise when the brain does not develop as expected. Sometimes, far back on day 23 of embryonic development, the front of the neural tube fails to close. The cerebral hemispheres and the skull around them never develop, and the child is born anencephalic, literally "without a brain," although the brain stem may be well formed. An anencephalic child is either stillborn or dies within a few days after birth.

Sometimes, in a condition called microcephaly, the brain is abnormally small, with a weight as low as 25% of normal. This condition can be caused by hereditary genetic problems that affect the developing brain. It can also happen when the normal development of the brain is disrupted by an infection, particularly rubella (German measles), toxoplasmosis (a parasite of cats), or syphilis. The most severe form of microcephaly is genetically inherited, and may cause severe mental retardation.

When the brain's intellectual functions fall below certain levels on standard IQ tests, an individual may be classified as mentally retarded. Using standard IQ measurements, over 90% of people classified as mentally retarded are designated as borderline or mildly retarded, without severe handicaps. In most of these individuals, medical evaluations have not found evidence of brain defects. The whole picture of mental retardation is complicated by the limits of our instruments, since IQ tests clearly do not measure all important intellectual functions. Specifically, they do not include evaluations of social skills or the ability to adapt to a changing environment.

In some cases, the brain may have an abnormally short attention span and may have trouble learning; its actions are impulsive, restless, excessive, "hyperactive." This problem has been called by different names, including attention deficit disorder, attention deficit hyperactivity disorder, and hyperactive syndrome. It is found in up to 10% of school children, mostly boys, and its cause is unknown. And there are controversies, since some specialists believe that the symptoms attributed to attention deficit disorder are not in fact due to just one disorder, but several, with different etiologies. Currently, researchers are investigating the role of hereditary factors, prenatal developmental problems, and psychosocial factors in the development of these symptoms. Some studies are focusing on abnormalities in the frontal lobes, especially problems in blood flow, abnormal levels of of certain neurotransmitters, or abnormalities in the receptors for those neurotransmitters.

Hyperactive children may also have learning disabilities, but many children with learning disabilities are *not* hyperactive. And not all children with diagnosed attention deficit disorder are hyperactive either.

Stimulant medications have been used successfully in treating children diagnosed as having attention deficit disorder. But some doctors have concerns about the overuse of these drugs, and they are beginning to investigate other types of therapy to supplement or replace medication.

The Growing Brain

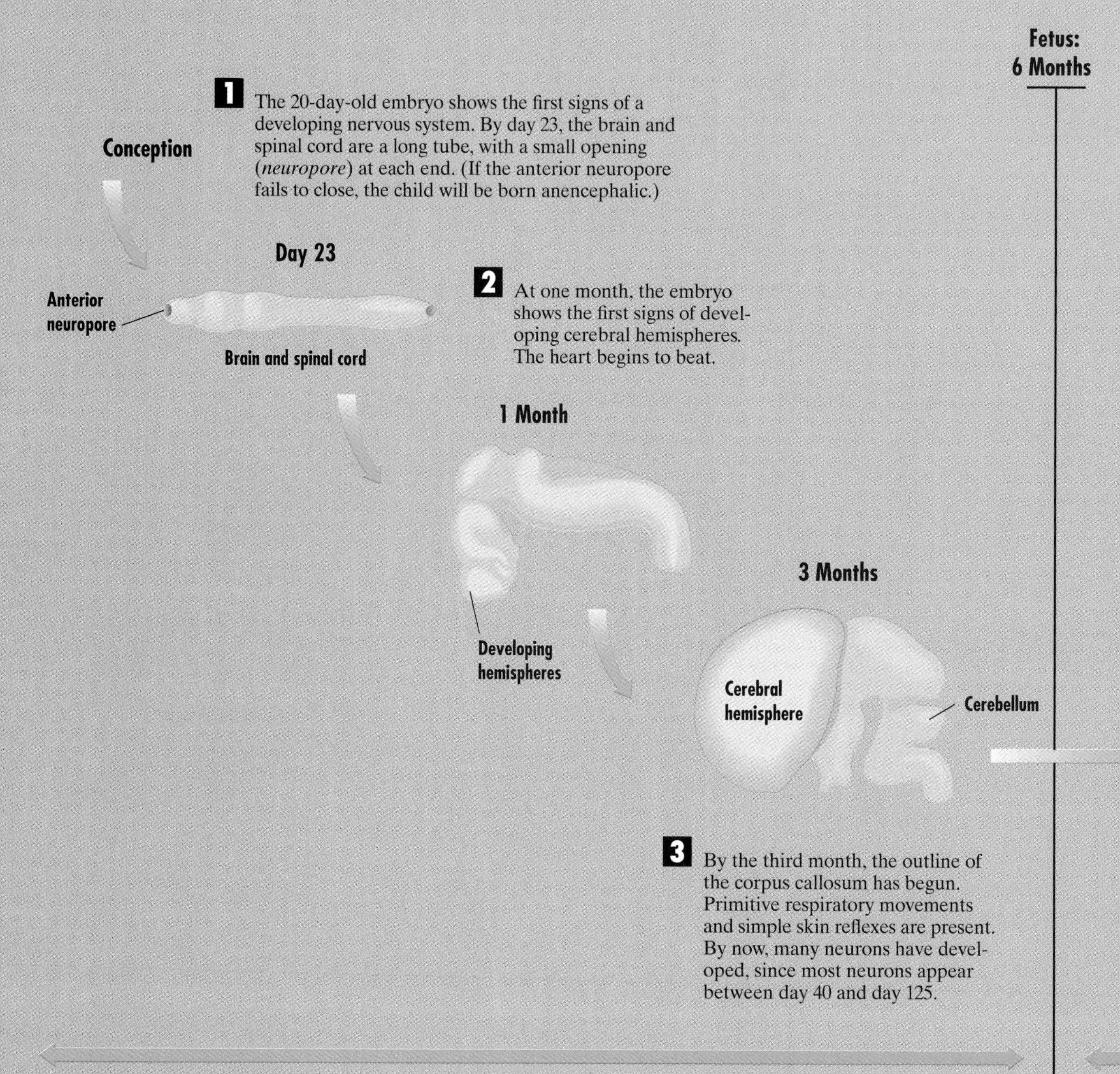

1 The 20-day-old embryo shows the first signs of a developing nervous system. By day 23, the brain and spinal cord are a long tube, with a small opening (*neuropore*) at each end. (If the anterior neuropore fails to close, the child will be born anencephalic.)

2 At one month, the embryo shows the first signs of developing cerebral hemispheres. The heart begins to beat.

3 By the third month, the outline of the corpus callosum has begun. Primitive respiratory movements and simple skin reflexes are present. By now, many neurons have developed, since most neurons appear between day 40 and day 125.

4 **Developmental Problems** Abnormal influences within the first six months after conception can cause very obvious problems in brain structure and can decrease the total number of neurons.

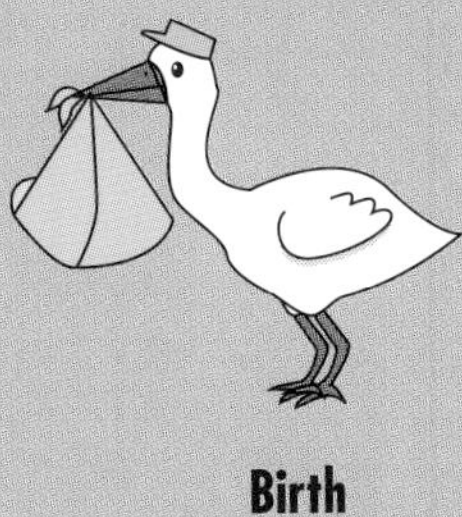

Birth

7 At birth, the brain is about 30% of adult size. Its major fissures are visible, along with a few prominent sulci and gyri. The stimulus of cold air on the skin, together with increasing carbon dioxide and decreasing oxygen concentrations in the blood, combine to activate the brain's respiratory center—the child takes his or her first breath. Hypothalamic control of body temperature is poor for the first few days of life.

1 Year Old

2 Years Old

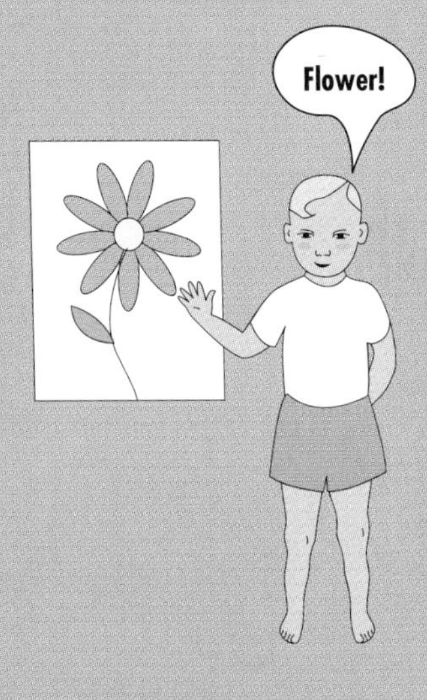

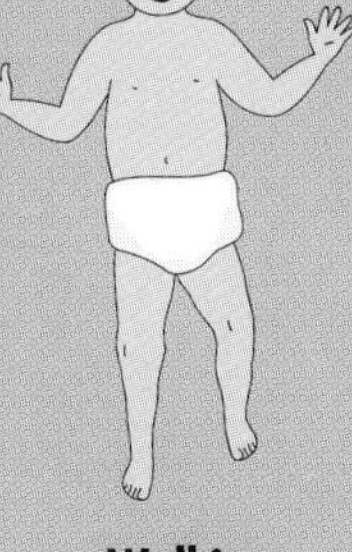

Sitting: 6–7 Months

Walking: 11–12 Months

8 During the first year of life, myelin is deposited to complete the fatty coating around the major tracts of white matter. The child sits, stands, and walks, indicating that these neural pathways are functionally complete. At the end of this first year, the brain is about 55% of adult size.

9 During the second year, the child climbs steps, names pictures of objects, and can speak in simple sentences (subject-verb-object). At the end of the second year, the brain is about 80% of adult size.

7 Months

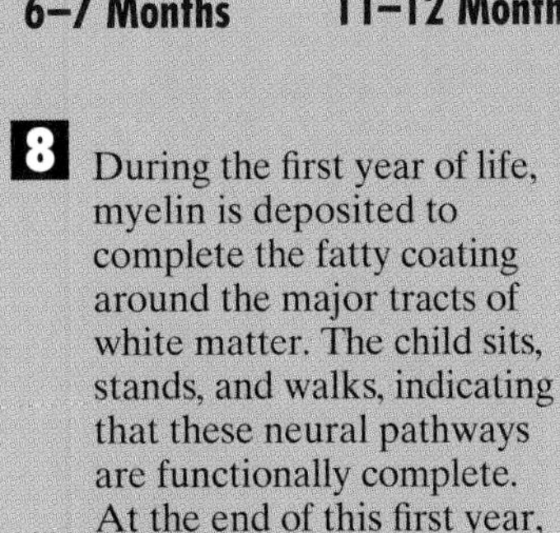

5 By six months, the outline of the corpus callosum is complete, but its fibers have no myelin coating. By six to seven months, the neural mechanisms that regulate the digestive system can function as well as in a newborn.

6 **Developmental Problems**
Abnormal influences that occur after the sixth month can cause more subtle changes in brain structure. The number of dendrites may decrease, or the formation of myelin around axons may be disrupted.

The Learning Brain

1 When a specific pattern of synapses is transmitted across a specific sequence of neurons, over and over again, the sequence becomes easier to repeat. Microscopic physical changes happen in the neurons involved. These changes form the basis for learning and memory.

2 For learning to happen, the axons and dendrites of neurons must be close enough to make synapses. Before birth, a neuron's position is determined by genetic factors and by chemical factors in the brain's environment that draw specific neurons to the same place and make them stick together. Neurons reach their position in the cortex of the developing embryo by sliding along the neuroglia, using them as guides.

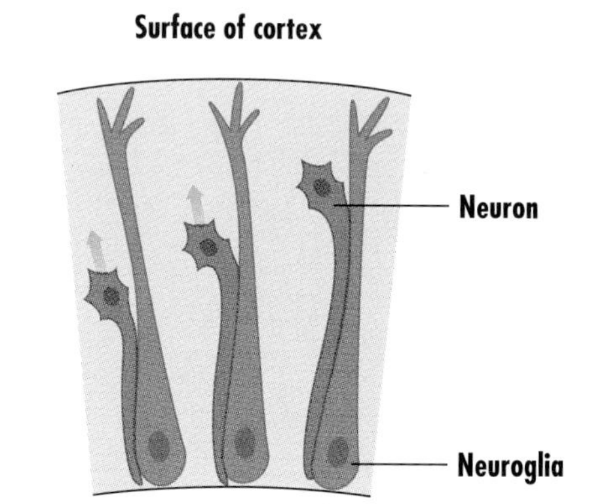

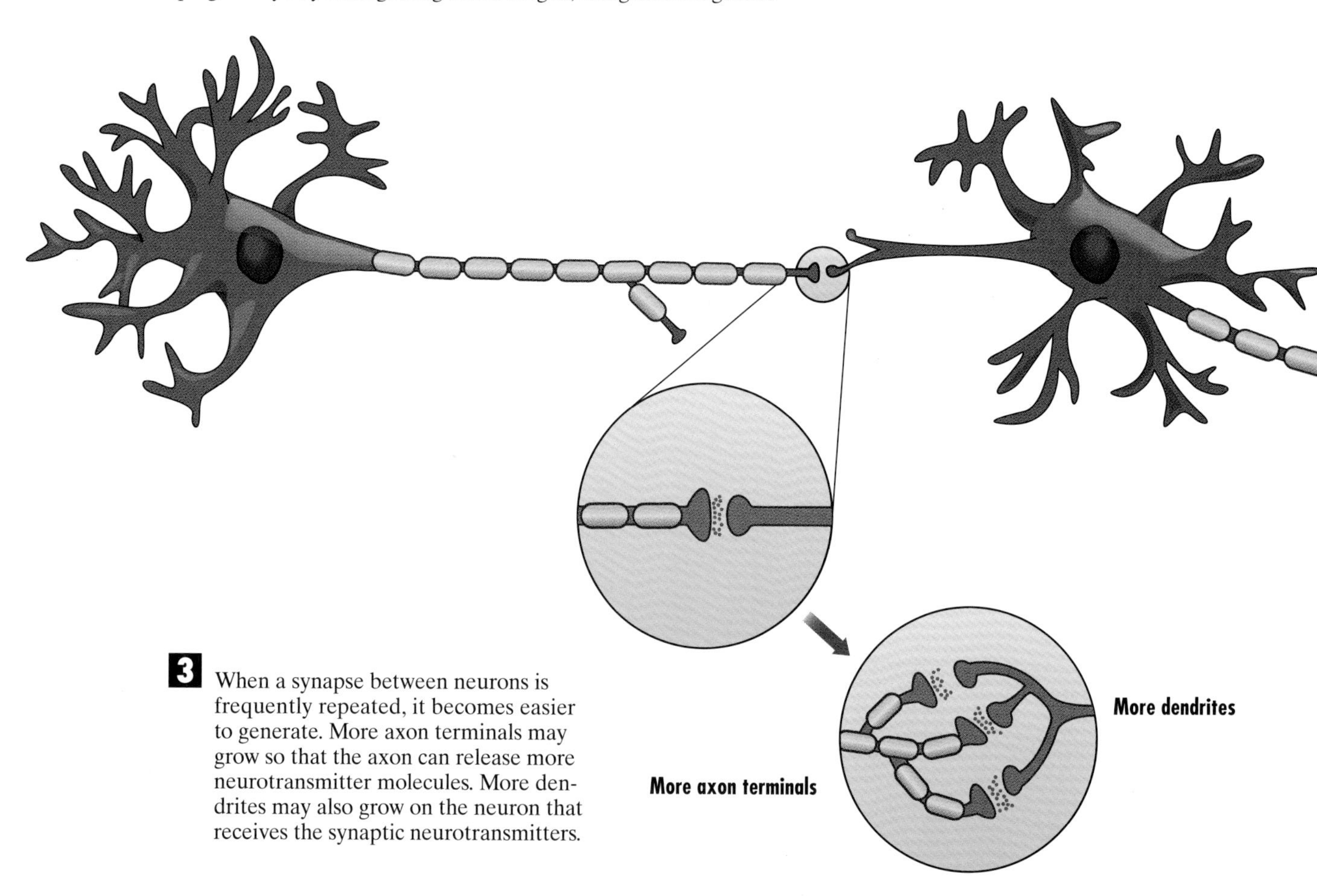

3 When a synapse between neurons is frequently repeated, it becomes easier to generate. More axon terminals may grow so that the axon can release more neurotransmitter molecules. More dendrites may also grow on the neuron that receives the synaptic neurotransmitters.

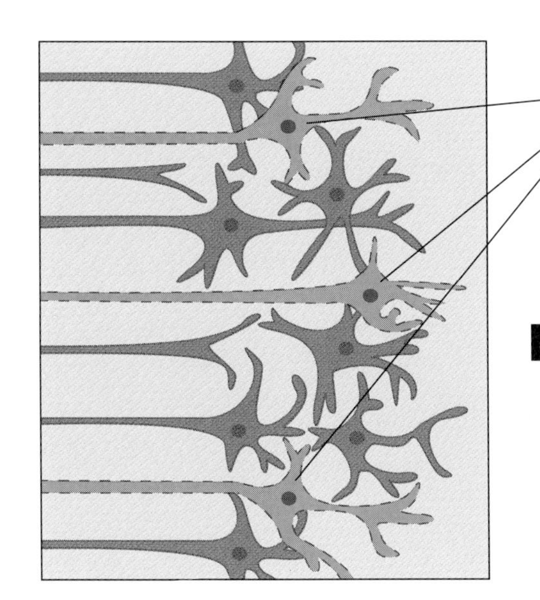

6 Neurons can wither if they are rarely used. Especially in early childhood, neurons that are never stimulated seem to just disappear. In this way, the electrical activity of nerve impulses sculpts the developing nervous system to fit the stimulation of its specific environment. Throughout life, learning keeps the brain healthy. An environment that is rich in sensory and intellectual stimulation can keep neurons active, make them grow larger, and increase the numbers of their axons and dendrites.

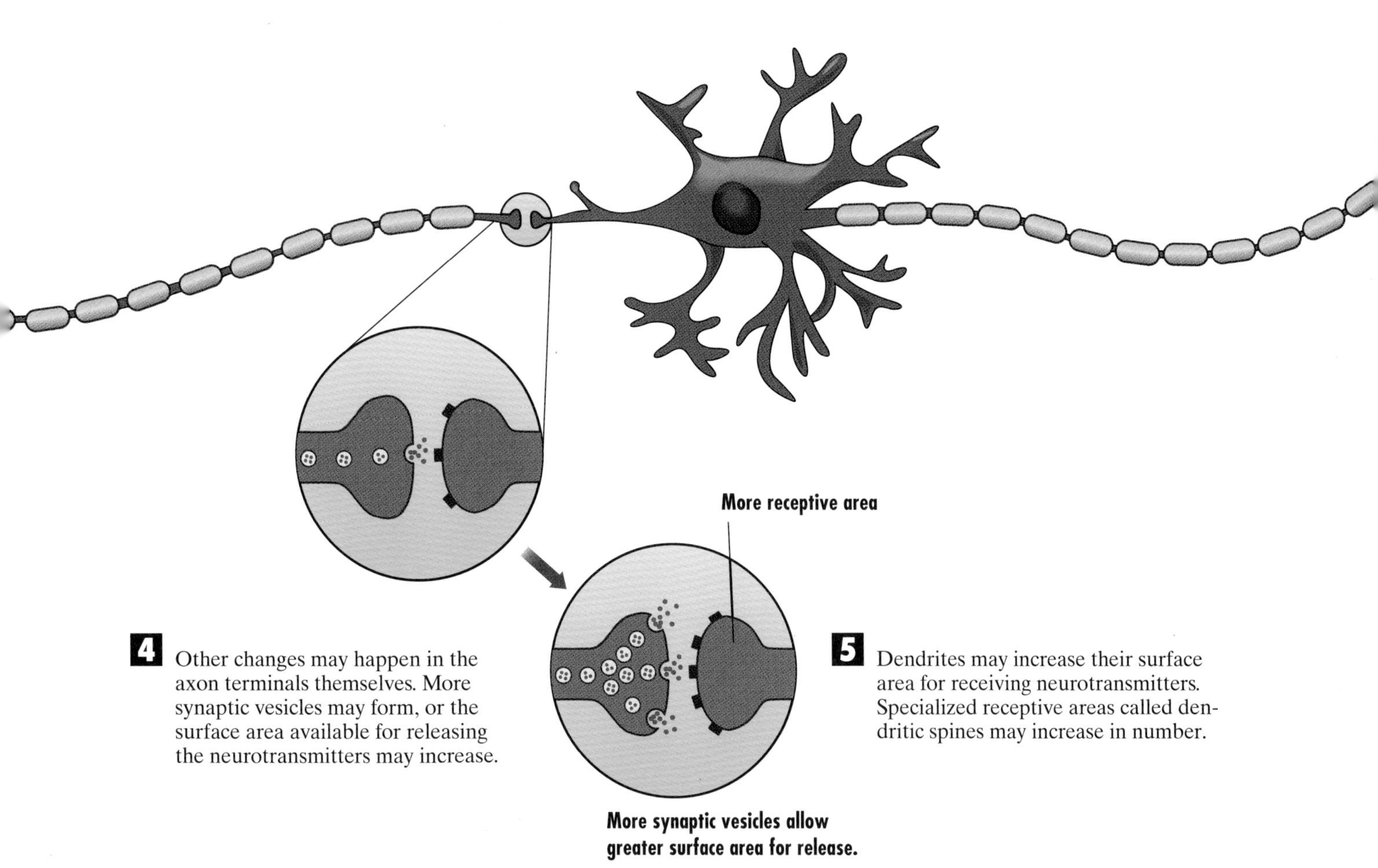

4 Other changes may happen in the axon terminals themselves. More synaptic vesicles may form, or the surface area available for releasing the neurotransmitters may increase.

5 Dendrites may increase their surface area for receiving neurotransmitters. Specialized receptive areas called dendritic spines may increase in number.

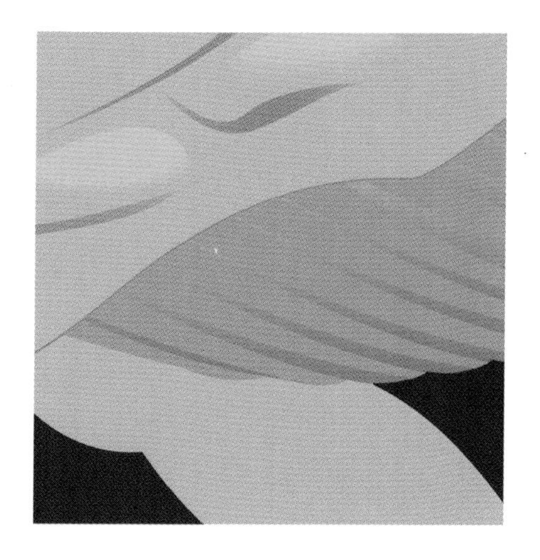

The Aging Brain
Lengthening Shadows

IN OUR HUMAN WORLD, we are accustomed to the lengthening shadows as a day passes. They are natural signs, not frightening omens. The brain, too, has its lengthening shadows, certain consistent signs that appear as the neuron population ages. And these are natural signs as well.

After middle age, the weight of the average brain tends to decrease and its blood flow may drop by 20%. Some neurons die, and those that remain alive may conduct their nerve impulses more slowly. The number of nerve fibers may decrease by more than one-third. As the ventricles enlarge and the trenchlike sulci widen, the whole neural world may shrink slightly. Brain metabolism may slow up to 16%.

Perhaps most noticeably, the senses may seem less sharp. The eyes may have some difficulty seeing objects close up, and the pupils may appear smaller and not as quick in their reaction to light. Hearing may be less acute, and the sense of smell may diminish. The taste of food may seem rather bland as more than half of the taste buds disappear.

Movement may become more or less difficult, depending on the interaction between aging muscles, joints, and nerves. There may be changes in stance and gait, as well as a greater tendency toward vertigo. Up to 30% of the spinal cord's motor neurons may die, causing muscles to become thinner and muscle power to decrease. The hand grip may be only 45% as strong as it was before, and the quick reflexes of youth will probably slow down.

Not all of these signs are found in all people, but most are fairly consistent with an average aging brain. Of course, on an individual basis, different brains do age differently, depending on their inherited genes and their life experiences. In a person with chronic heart or lung disease, for example, the brain may have endured prolonged periods of poor oxygen supply. In a person with a history of violence, the brain may have suffered through a lifetime of repeated traumas. Because the brain is so dependent on the rest of the body, it is difficult to isolate the affects of age on the brain without considering the neural implications of problems in other body organs. And because the brain spends its entire life depending on other body organs for its resources, this dependency makes the brain a second victim if one of these organ systems malfunctions or fails.

As the brain ages, it may show some mild memory problems, especially regarding proper names and recent events. But when an older person's memory becomes severely impaired, the brain may be suffering from Alzheimer's disease.

Scientists once thought that Alzheimer's disease was merely an unusually advanced or premature senile change, but this is no longer so. In Alzheimer's disease there is a *selective* loss of neurons, together with an abnormal accumulation of amyloid protein (amyloid plaques) and the formation of fibrous structures called neurofibrillary tangles. These microscopic changes affect cortical areas that process information in the frontal, temporal, and parietal lobes, together with the hippocampus and areas of the limbic system. Neurons in the primary sensory, motor, auditory, and visual areas are usually spared.

Alzheimer's disease typically begins with an insidious loss of memory and progresses to affect speech, comprehension, calculation, and orientation. Sight, hearing, sensation, and reflexes are usually normal. Gait may also be normal but can deteriorate as the disease progresses. Psychiatric disturbances, like depression and disruptive behavior (wandering and repetitive manipulation of objects), may also be seen.

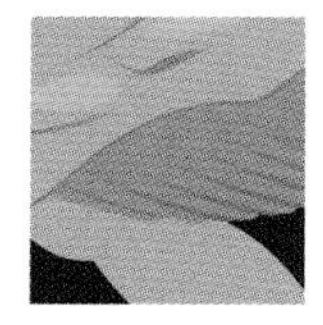

The diagnosis of Alzheimer's disease can be made by neuroradiological scans, often called PET or SPECT scans. SPECT scans may show a decreased metabolism in the temporal and parietal areas of the cerebral cortex.

There is currently no therapy to change the final course of Alzheimer's disease, but new drugs that enhance the brain's use of the neurotransmitter acetylcholine have been effective in relieving some of the symptoms. Antioxidants, including vitamins E, C, and A (beta-carotene), are also being tested. These compounds may help protect the body against damage caused by free radicals, toxic compounds that accumulate in the body as a result of complex oxygen reactions. There is evidence, too, that people who remain intellectually active by interacting with a stimulating environment can help delay or decrease the effects of Alzheimer's disease.

With each day of its lifetime, the brain loses more and more neurons, and there is no magic formula to prevent this loss. Even the living neurons of the aging brain seem to undergo changes in their internal chemicals that slow down their vital chemistry. Scientists are now looking at different ways to prevent damage to the neuron's internal enzyme systems. Until their efforts produce new (and proven) ways to slow the brain's aging, a practical look at what kills a neuron can lead to some guidelines for saving one.

Trauma. Neurons can die if they are physically hurt, and previous head injury may be a risk factor for Alzheimer's disease and for epilepsy. A blow to the head can cause a double brain injury as the brain ricochets against the opposite side of the skull wall.

Practical measures for prevention of head injuries include air bags and seat belts in cars, head gear appropriate for contact sports, and helmets for those who skate or ride bicycles or motorcycles.

Starvation and asphyxiation. Neurons need food and oxygen. Starvation diets and smoking do not provide what the brain needs. People who have problems involving the heart, lungs, or liver can indirectly help the brain by following medical advice about diet and medication. Any new drug therapy or new combination of drugs should be checked for side effects that target the brain. This is especially true in the elderly, where the most common cause of confusion is not a physical illness, but a problem related to medication.

Toxins. Harmful substances that disturb the brain's natural environment should be avoided. Drugs that make the brain hallucinate, convulse, tremble, or lose consciousness also have the potential to kill neurons. And a dead neuron is dead forever.

Infections. The brain is an organ that can be attacked by bacteria and viruses. High fevers, especially if accompanied by convulsions, changes in vision, headache, or a stiff neck, require medical attention.

Lethargy. There is microscopic evidence that "exercising" the brain is good for neurons. Involved, intellectually active individuals who find stimulation in their environments appear to have larger, healthier neurons with more axons and dendrites. Although some neurons are lost with age, those that remain are gifted with a rich synaptic history. A lifetime of learning and sensory experience is the priceless treasure within every "senior" brain. And because learning never has to stop, many older people choose to pursue new vocations, even attend college, after they retire.

Brain functions that are used in daily life, including comprehension and imagination, often are as high in older people as in young adults. And in some studies, older people tested even higher in reasoning and judgment as they passed from their mid-60s to their mid-70s and mid-80s.

Someday we may be able to postpone, prevent, or even reverse the physical changes of aging in the brain. As research continues, scientists are exploring antioxidants, stress-reduction techniques, and even gene therapy, as ways to limit the effects of time on the brain.

The Brain Ages: Some Consistent Signs

1 As the brain ages it undergoes a number of global changes. Its sulci and ventricles widen. Between midlife and death, its weight may decrease by 15%, and its blood flow by 20%. Brain metabolism may be about 16% slower. Changes in the regulatory centers of the hypothalamus may affect the whole body. For example, a decreased drive for thirst and a less sensitive response to low levels of body water may increase the risk of dehydration.

Motor

Sensory

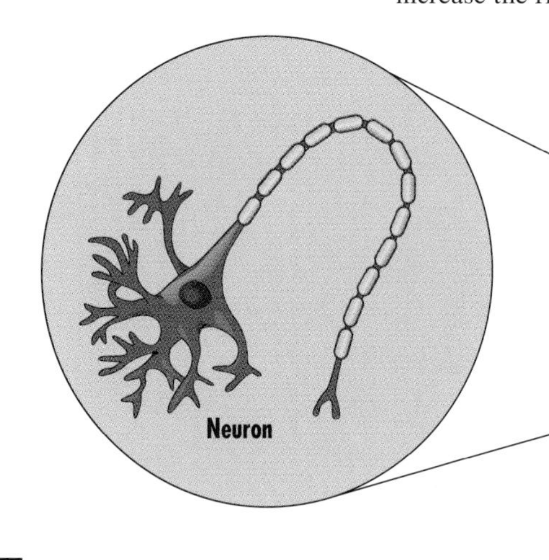

2 As neurons age, some die. Those that remain alive may be 10% slower in conducting nerve impulses. The number of nerve fibers may decrease by over one-third.

3 The sense of smell (olfactory nerves) diminishes.

Olfactory nerve

4 Vision for nearby objects becomes less acute. Pupils become smaller and react more slowly to light. The ability to look upward may diminish.

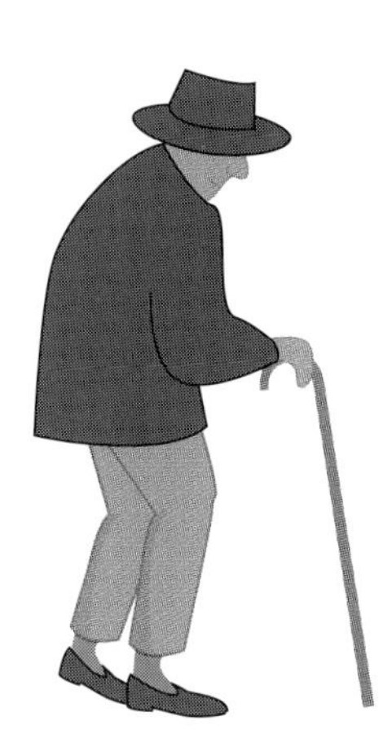

5 Movement of muscles may become difficult, and muscle power may decrease. Strength of hand grip may diminish by 45%. Walking may be easier if short steps are used.

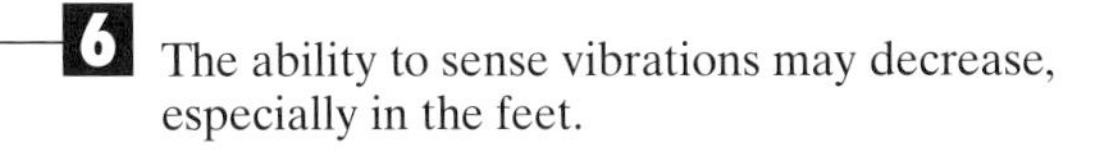

6 The ability to sense vibrations may decrease, especially in the feet.

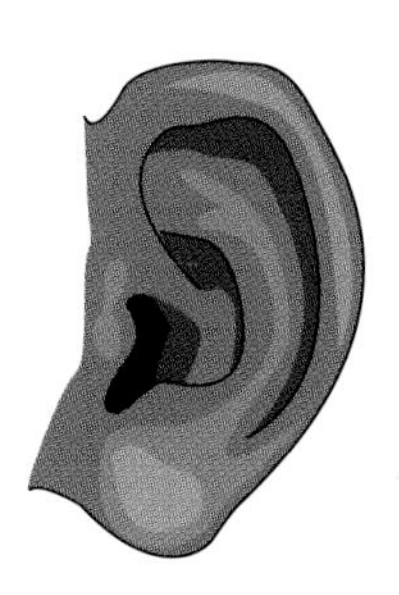

7 Hearing loss, especially of higher-frequency sounds, can happen because of loss of hair cells in the inner ear. Hardening of the arteries can diminish blood supply to the auditory nerve and to the brain's deep auditory pathways, causing problems in localizing sounds, most noticeably in a noisy room.

8 The body becomes less agile and balance becomes more difficult. There may be a greater tendency toward vertigo.

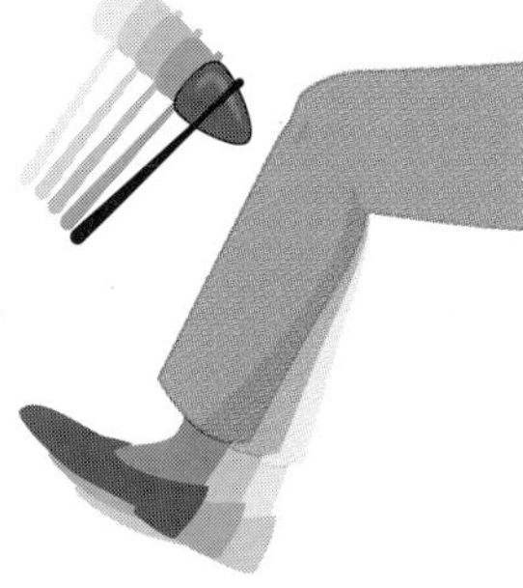

9 Up to 30% of the spinal cord's motor neurons may die between age 60 and 90. Muscles, especially leg muscles, become thinner as their motor neurons die. The knee-jerk and many other reflexes diminish.

PART

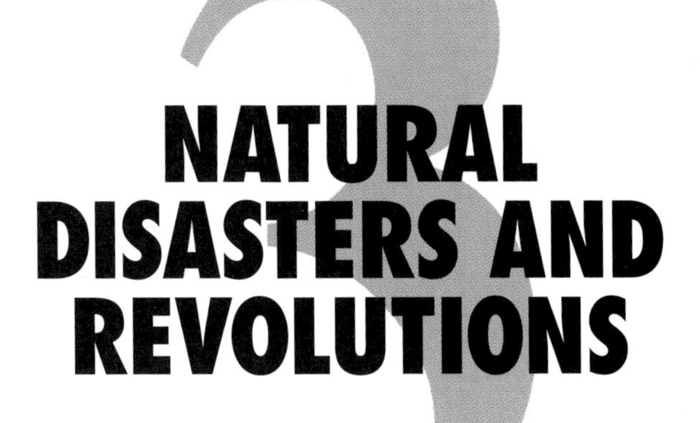

NATURAL DISASTERS AND REVOLUTIONS

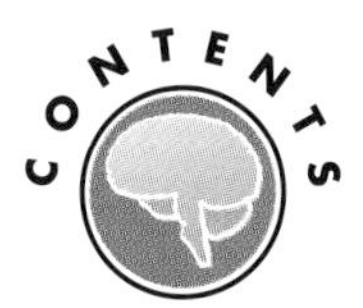

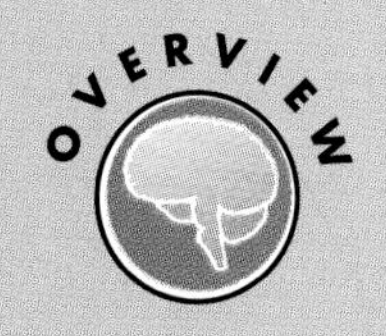
OVERVIEW

THE HEALTHY BRAIN is usually a peaceful and busy world where the population of neurons remains orderly and the environment is delicately balanced. Yet there are times when, in spite of all its protective and regulatory mechanisms, the brain becomes as vulnerable as any other world to threats from without or within.

Just as the human world has social upheavals and natural disasters, the brain has seizures, headaches, and psychiatric problems. We may see these phenomena as illnesses in themselves, or they may form complex signs of overlapping problems. A severe headache, for example, may follow a seizure, or psychiatric symptoms may signal a rare form of epilepsy. These phenomena may also serve as neural alarms, warning about a toxin or disease elsewhere in the body.

In Part 3 of this book we examine how seizures, headaches, and psychiatric problems arise in the brain, and how the brain is attacked by tumors, toxins, and HIV.

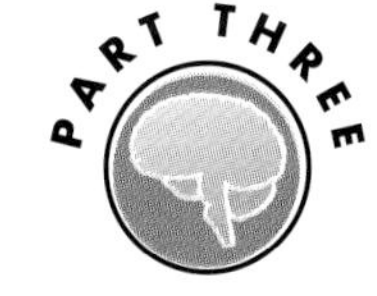

We begin by looking at how neurons may become unstable and fire abnormally, causing waves of seizure activity through the brain. Seizures can result in a wide range of disordered sensations and uncontrolled muscle movements, even loss of consciousness and death.

Next, we examine how neuron behavior influences psychiatric illness and why researchers believe that many psychiatric problems are disorders caused by abnormal communications between neurons. We will see that these illnesses have a biological basis as well as a behavioral one.

We explore how, apart from the normal neuron population, bizarre and dangerous groups of cells may arise in the brain. These abnormal cell populations may grow uncontrollably and aggressively. They may form gliomas and other potentially deadly types of brain tumors. We will discover how "foreign" cancers, from the lung, breast, skin, and elsewhere, are capable of invading the brain as well.

We next examine the many forms of headache, and how a headache can be another problem with a "foreign" origin, beginning in a sinus infection or in muscle spasms around the head. We'll learn about headaches that warn of threats much closer to the brain, threats such as meningitis or bleeding from a major blood vessel.

Finally, we investigate the mechanisms by which toxins and HIV, both extreme forms of foreign assault, can violate the delicate ecology of the brain.

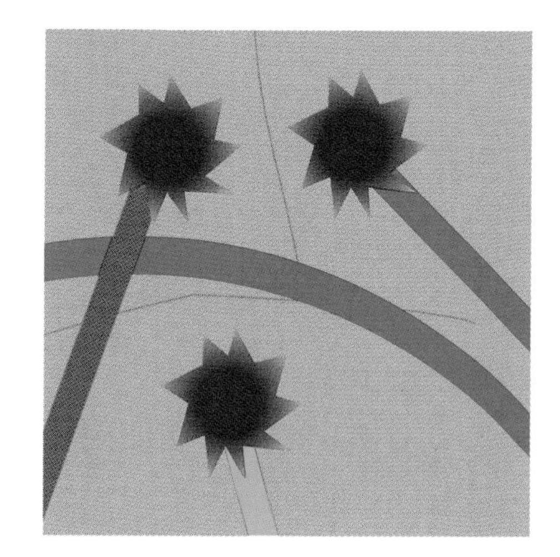

Seizures and Epilepsy
Neural Uprisings

OFTEN IN HUMAN HISTORY, people have left their quiet everyday work to unite in revolution or war. Upheaval has been followed by resolution and reconstruction, with the eventual return of normal life. In the brain, too, neurons can leave their peaceful random firing patterns and unite to produce dramatic, abnormal, synchronized nerve impulses called seizures.

The brain has seizures for different reasons. In newborn children, seizures are often caused by hypoxia or injury to the brain at birth, by infection, or by abnormalities of blood chemistry (decreased levels of blood sugar, calcium, or magnesium). Later in life, seizures are more likely to be part of the brain's reaction to a tumor, blood vessel problem, or toxic drug. In many cases they are idiopathic, of unknown origin. When seizures are chronic and recurrent, the brain is described as suffering from epilepsy.

Not all seizures are the same. Some involve the entire brain, while others involve only part. Some last only a few seconds and are barely noticeable, while others last much longer and cause a very obvious loss of consciousness.

When a seizure begins all over the cortex at once, it is called a primary generalized seizure. A primary generalized seizure may be either of the grand mal or petit mal type. In a *grand mal* seizure, abnormal nerve impulses spread bilaterally across the corpus callosum to involve the entire cerebral cortex symmetrically. The brain is overwhelmed by neuron activity and loses consciousness. Muscles everywhere in the body contract at once, and the person falls to the ground, stops breathing, and turns blue. This initial sustained muscle contraction is followed by a series of shorter rhythmic muscle contractions. The seizure episode lasts for more than a minute, and is followed by a period of relaxation and eventual recovery.

In the *petit mal* type of primary generalized seizure, the episode also involves the entire cerebral cortex, but it lasts only a few seconds. The loss of consciousness is so brief that the person usually doesn't change position, but remains sitting or standing just as before. The only obvious sign of a petite mal seizure may be a blinking of the eyes or a brief rhythmic movement of an extremity.

In *partial (focal) seizures,* the abnormal discharge of neurons begins in a specific and usually identifiable location in the brain called a seizure focus. The abnormal activity of neurons in the seizure focus produces symptoms that correspond to the area of the brain where the focus is located. A seizure focus in the frontal lobe's motor area, for example, could cause abnormal muscle movements as a symptom of seizure activity, while a focus in the temporal lobe might cause emotional symptoms, such as fear or rage. (This would involve the temporal lobe's limbic structures. For more on the limbic system, see Chapter 8.)

Often, the brain's natural inhibitory defense systems can limit the turmoil of partial seizures to a small area of the brain. But at other times, the partial seizure activity can recruit neighboring neurons into its abnormal pattern. The partial seizure can spread beyond the area of the seizure focus to include wider areas of the brain. This can cause alterations in the state of consciousness and may even result in bizarre behavior that the person will not recall when the seizure ends.

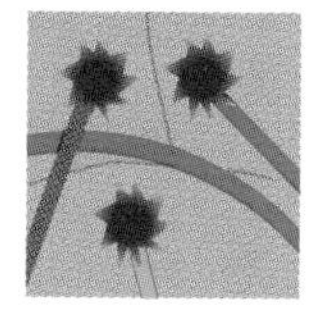

When drugs, infection, or abnormalities in blood chemistry are the underlying problems causing seizures, it is often possible to calm the seizure activity by treating the underlying problem. In cases of idiopathic seizures, the situation is more complex, since the problem lies somewhere in the microscopic anatomy or physiology of the neurons themselves. For some reason, these neurons seem to be inherently unstable. They are a vulnerable population that responds to many different stimuli by triggering a seizure.

Seizures are sometimes caused by a localized and limited problem in the brain, such as a tumor, cyst, or abscess. Surgical removal of the local problem will often stop the seizures or make them easier to control with medication.

As much as 2% of the population of the United States is currently living with some form of recurrent seizures—some form of epilepsy. The diagnosis of epilepsy may have a serious impact on various aspects of a person's life, including choice of job and ability to drive a car. Grand mal seizures, in particular, can strike without warning, causing head injury and fractured bones from falls.

Researchers are trying to understand the mechanisms behind seizures in order to develop better medications to prevent them. Ideally, such medications could raise the threshold of neurons to make them less "excitable" or could intensify the inhibitory influences between neurons to keep abnormal nerve impulses from spreading across synapses. Currently available medications such as phenytoin, carbamazepine, phenobarbital, and valproic acid are effective against grand mal seizures, but they have potentially dangerous side effects, especially at higher doses. Several new medications that claim fewer side effects are now coming onto the market, but their success remains to be seen.

Rarely, generalized seizures follow one another without allowing the person to regain consciousness. This is status epilepticus, a life-threatening medical emergency, that causes death in about 10% of patients. It is treated by intravenous medications, together with protective measures to keep the airways open and to prevent injury to the head and tongue.

Types of Seizures: Focus and Spread

1 In the normal waking brain, each neuron does it own work, firing nerve impulses as needed to help the brain perform the activities of daily life. The firing pattern appears random but really reflects the changing requirements of the brain for the services of different neurons at different times.

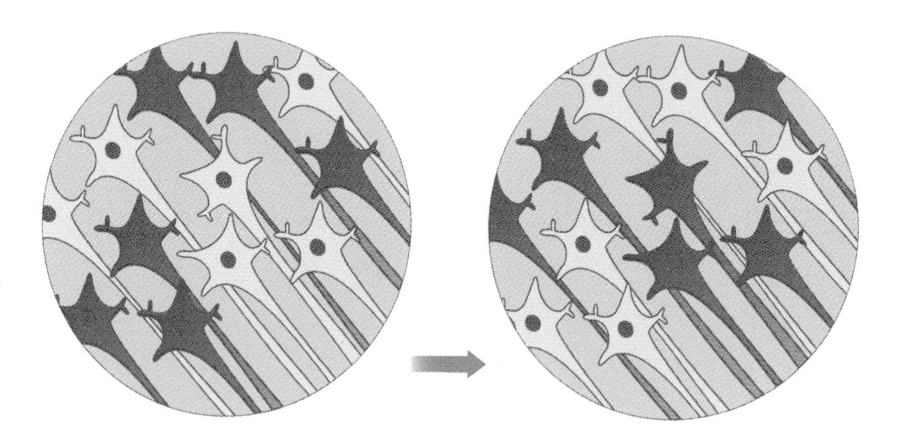

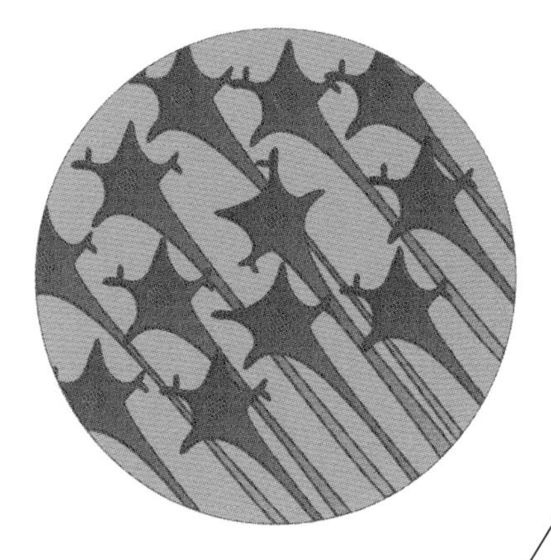

2 In a seizure focus, inherently unstable neurons lose their haphazard firing pattern and unite to fire all at once, producing synchronized, rhythmic nerve impulses.

Partial (Focal) Seizures

3 In a partial (focal) seizure, the location of the seizure focus determines the symptoms of the seizure. A seizure focus in the motor area of the frontal lobe may produce involuntary movements, while a temporal lobe seizure focus may produce emotional symptoms or memory disturbances like déjà vu. A seizure focus in any sensory area may cause sensory hallucinations of false smells, sights, or sounds. Partial seizures often remain localized to one area of the brain, but they can spread. They may rarely cause altered or impaired consciousness, along with unusual behavior that is not remembered when the seizure ends.

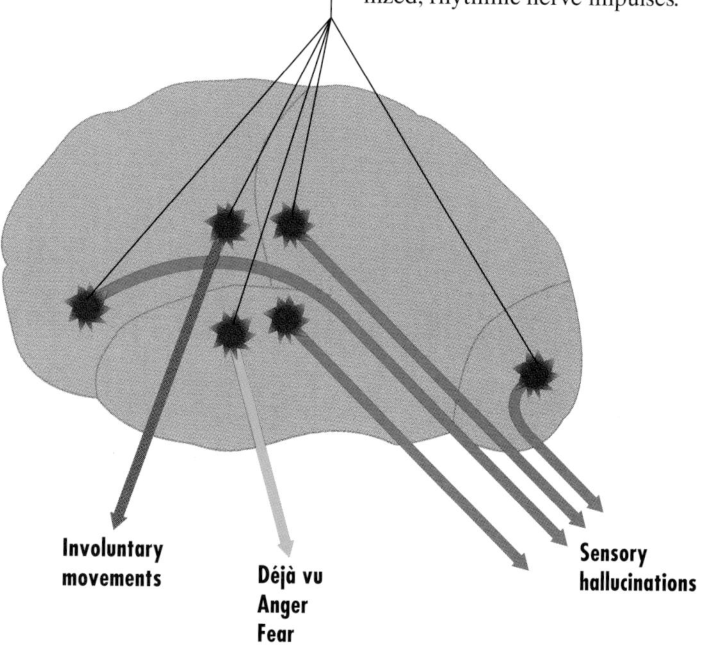

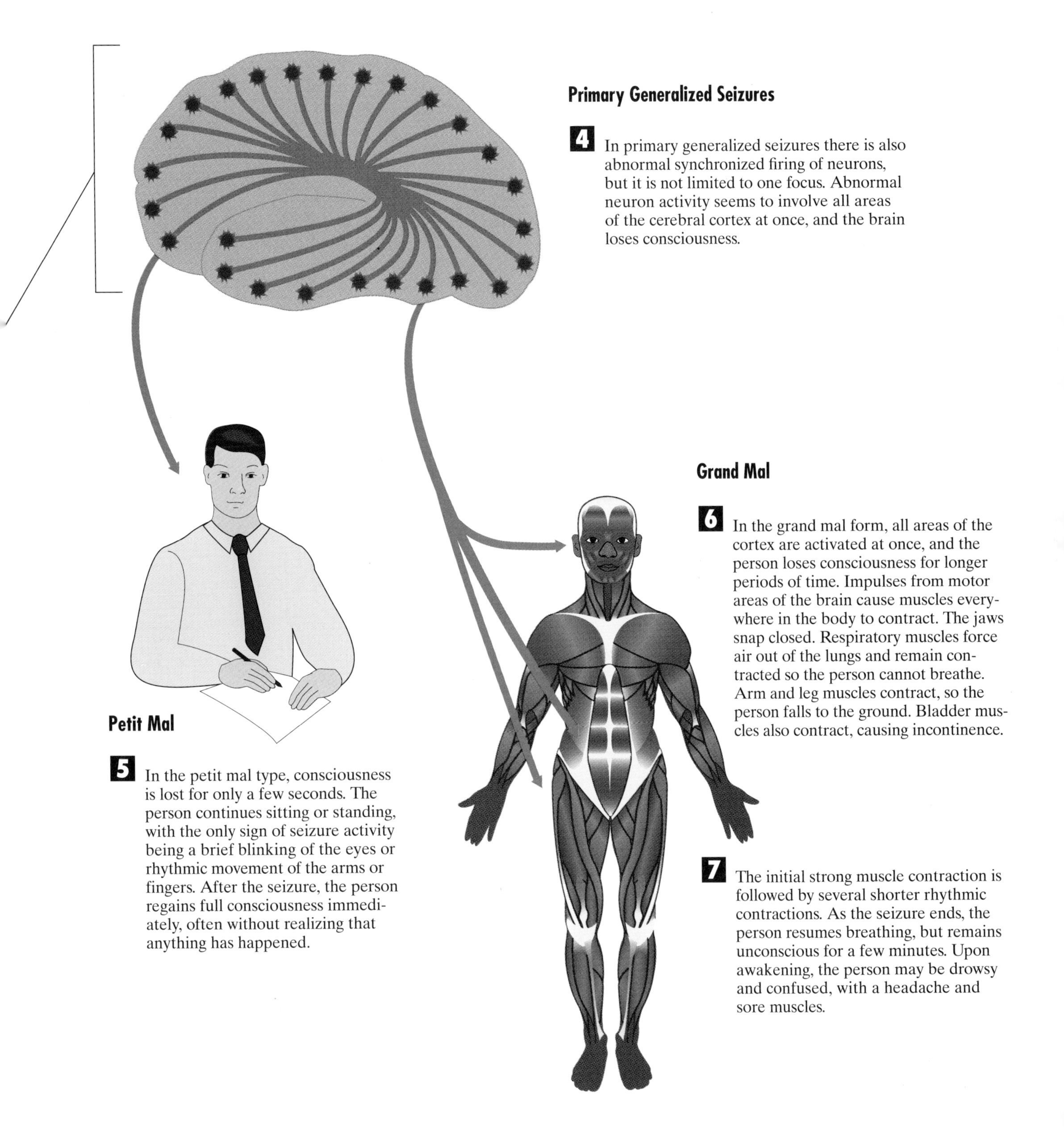

Primary Generalized Seizures

4 In primary generalized seizures there is also abnormal synchronized firing of neurons, but it is not limited to one focus. Abnormal neuron activity seems to involve all areas of the cerebral cortex at once, and the brain loses consciousness.

Petit Mal

5 In the petit mal type, consciousness is lost for only a few seconds. The person continues sitting or standing, with the only sign of seizure activity being a brief blinking of the eyes or rhythmic movement of the arms or fingers. After the seizure, the person regains full consciousness immediately, often without realizing that anything has happened.

Grand Mal

6 In the grand mal form, all areas of the cortex are activated at once, and the person loses consciousness for longer periods of time. Impulses from motor areas of the brain cause muscles everywhere in the body to contract. The jaws snap closed. Respiratory muscles force air out of the lungs and remain contracted so the person cannot breathe. Arm and leg muscles contract, so the person falls to the ground. Bladder muscles also contract, causing incontinence.

7 The initial strong muscle contraction is followed by several shorter rhythmic contractions. As the seizure ends, the person resumes breathing, but remains unconscious for a few minutes. Upon awakening, the person may be drowsy and confused, with a headache and sore muscles.

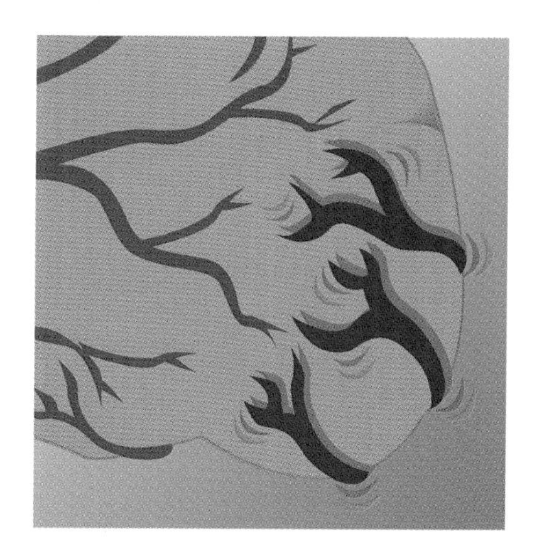

Headaches

Neural Alarms, False and True

WHEN SIRENS WAKE US on a hot summer night, their sound triggers a series of automatic questions in our minds. Where is the problem and how bad is it? Are there other indications of danger nearby—gunshots, screams, or the smell of smoke? In the brain, headaches are much like those sirens in the night. They may mean nothing, or they may mean imminent danger. It all depends on their location, intensity, and associated symptoms.

The brain, which feels pain for the entire body, has a limited capacity for feeling pain in areas closest to itself. Remarkably, the substance of the brain, and the skull around it, are not sensitive to pain. Only the skin and muscles around the skull feel pain, as do the eyes, the nose, the sinuses around the nose, and the membrane (periosteum) lining the inside of the skull. The brain's arteries, veins, venous sinuses (Chapter 3), and three of its cranial nerves (trigeminal, vagus, and glossopharyngeal) are also sensitive to pain.

What we call "headache" is produced by stimulating one of the select pain-sensitive structures in the head. For example, headaches result when arteries or veins are pulled, displaced, dilated, or distended. They also happen when cranial nerves are pulled, compressed, or inflamed. Trauma or spasm of facial or neck muscles can produce a headache, as can sinus infections.

After knowing which structures can possibly "hurt" near the brain, it is easier to group headaches into categories according to their location, intensity, and associated symptoms.

Tension headache is the most common type of chronic headache seen by doctors. The pain of tension headache may concentrate in the frontal or occipital area, and is often described as an aching, fullness, or pressure. Tension headache may be caused by sustained muscle spasms of the head and neck, but new research is focusing on the brain's blood vessels. Depression and anxiety are symptoms often associated with tension headache and, in some cases, antidepressants and anxiolytic (antianxiety) medications are prescribed.

Migraine headaches usually appear in adolescence. In *classic* (*neurologic*) *migraine*, a throbbing headache involves the frontal and temporal areas of one side of the head. Neurologic warning symptoms, called prodromata, appear before the headache begins and may include visual disturbances (sparkles or wavy lines), numbness, weakness, or vertigo. The headache itself may be associated with nausea and vomiting. In *common migraine*, the headache is similar to neurologic migraine, but without the prodromata.

The pain of migraine is probably caused by dilation (widening) of the arteries of the head and brain. Researchers are unsure of the exact mechanisms, but some are focusing on disturbances in nerves that regulate the diameter of the brain's blood vessels or on mechanisms involving the neurotransmitter serotonin.

Most authorities believe that migraine, especially classic migraine, may be hereditary. As treatment, aspirin or non-narcotic pain medications are sometimes sufficient, but severe attacks may require ergotamine, either alone or combined with caffeine. Ergotamine constricts widened arteries, returning them to a nearly normal diameter and stopping the headache pain. Propranolol and other drugs may be used as prevention. It may also be helpful to avoid alcohol, coffee, tea, chocolate, milk, or wheat products.

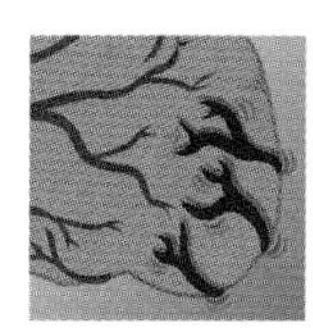

Cluster headaches usually afflict young adult males. Headache pain is intense, constant, and typically located around one eye. It begins within 1 to 2 hours after the patient falls asleep and is so severe that it awakens him. The headache only lasts for about 20 to 30 minutes, but it returns the next night, and every night afterwards, for periods (clusters) of weeks or months. Accompanying symptoms include tearing and redness of the eyes, runny nose, and flushed forehead or cheek. The exact cause of cluster headache is not known. Like migraine, cluster headaches can be treated with ergotamine. They can be prevented with prednisone.

Sinus headache accompanies sinus infection and is usually felt around the eyes or in the forehead. The skin in these areas may also be tender. The nose is blocked and there is a nasal discharge. Treatment includes antibiotics and nasal decongestants.

Headache of brain tumor is often a deep, bursting pain that may awaken the person in the middle of the night. The headache may be accompanied by unexpected and forceful vomiting. If the headache is one-sided (unilateral) it is almost always on the same side of the head as the tumor.

Common everyday headache does not usually require a visit to the doctor. These headaches are treated effectively by each of us at home, often with aspirin or acetaminophen. They may be due to fatigue, overwork, stress, too much smoking, drinking alcohol, or eating certain types of food.

Headache emergencies occur when the pain is unusually severe ("the worst headache I've ever had"), develops abruptly, and becomes intense over a short period of time. Causes include stroke and meningitis.

Stroke is the third leading cause of death in developed countries and affects 400,000 persons annually in the United States. Strokes are caused by sudden interruptions of the brain's blood flow, with subsequent death or injury of brain cells. Interruption of blood flow happens because of blockage or rupture of one of the brain's arteries.

A brain artery can be blocked either by a thrombus (a blood clot developing locally) or by an embolus (a blood clot or piece of debris floating in the bloodstream). Strokes caused by a thrombus or an embolus may cause headaches, but they also cause other important symptoms, such as weakness, paralysis, sensory impairment, and problems with speech or vision.

Headache that is sudden and severe is a common symptom of strokes caused by rupture of one of the brain's arteries, resulting in bleeding (hemorrhage) in the brain. This type of stroke is either due to hypertensive hemorrhage or to rupture of a saccular aneurysm or arteriovenous malformation.

Strokes from hypertensive hemorrhage usually occur in people with a history of high blood pressure. A blood vessel breaks and bleeds deep in the brain. There is severe headache and vomiting, often with loss of consciousness and coma.

Strokes due to ruptured blood vessel malformations may be caused by ruptured saccular aneurysms or arteriovenous malformations. Saccular aneurysms are berry-shaped swellings of a brain artery, which may rupture and bleed into the subarachnoid space of the brain (subarachnoid hemorrhage). This causes abrupt and severe headache, nausea and vomiting, and stiff neck. Arteriovenous malformations are abnormal tangled masses of small blood vessels. Ruptured arteriovenous malformations may also cause a subarachnoid hemorrhage.

Meningitis is inflammation of the meninges. Headache is an important symptom of meningitis caused by a bacterial or viral infection. It is usually associated with fever and other signs of infection, stiff neck, drowsiness, and sometimes confusion or seizures. Headache can be a symptom of many diverse medical problems including carbon monoxide poisoning, chronic lung disease, thyroid or adrenal problems, pituitary tumors, and anemia. It can also be a side effect of heart medications containing nitrates and of certain contraceptive medications.

Like a siren in the night, headache is only a warning sign, and knowing when to be alarmed depends upon prior headache experience and informed judgment.

Headache: Where the Head Feels Pain

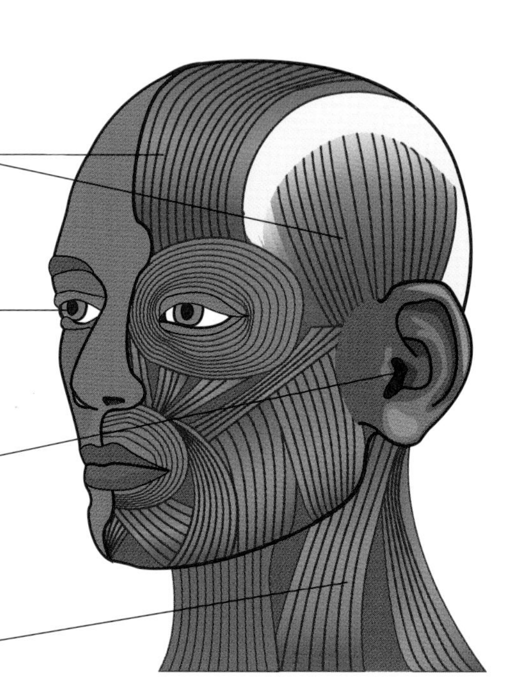

1 Sustained contraction of head muscles may cause some tension headaches. Also, squinting because of poor vision may strain forehead muscles and cause headache.

2 Eye problems, such as glaucoma, eye muscle imbalance, and astigmatism, can cause pain in the eye, or in the head around the eye.

3 Infection or pressure changes in the ear (especially during airplane flights) can cause pain in the ear or around it. A stroke blocking the vertebral artery can cause pain in back of the ear.

4 Problems in the muscles and joints of the neck can cause headache in the occipital area. Examples include arthritis and whiplash injuries.

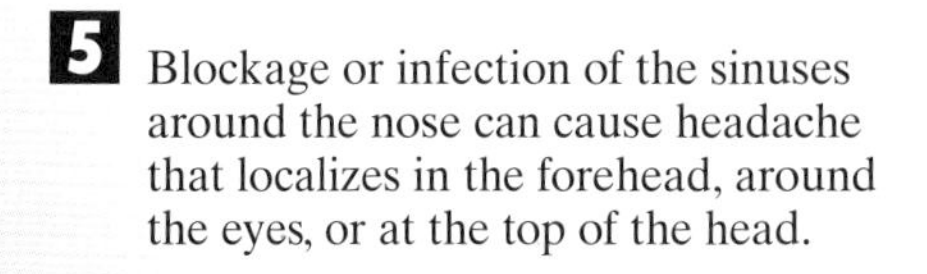

5 Blockage or infection of the sinuses around the nose can cause headache that localizes in the forehead, around the eyes, or at the top of the head.

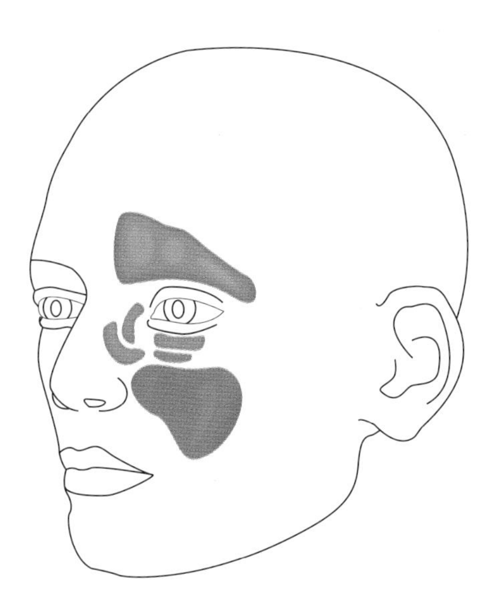

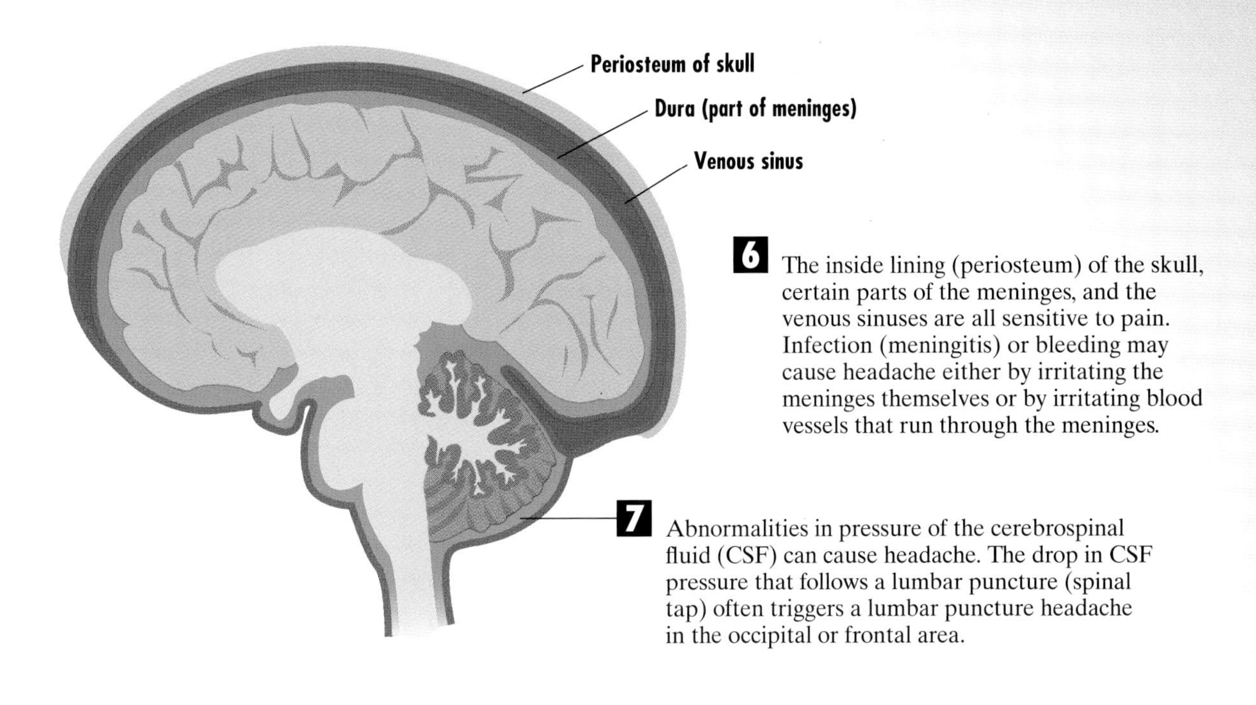

6 The inside lining (periosteum) of the skull, certain parts of the meninges, and the venous sinuses are all sensitive to pain. Infection (meningitis) or bleeding may cause headache either by irritating the meninges themselves or by irritating blood vessels that run through the meninges.

7 Abnormalities in pressure of the cerebrospinal fluid (CSF) can cause headache. The drop in CSF pressure that follows a lumbar puncture (spinal tap) often triggers a lumbar puncture headache in the occipital or frontal area.

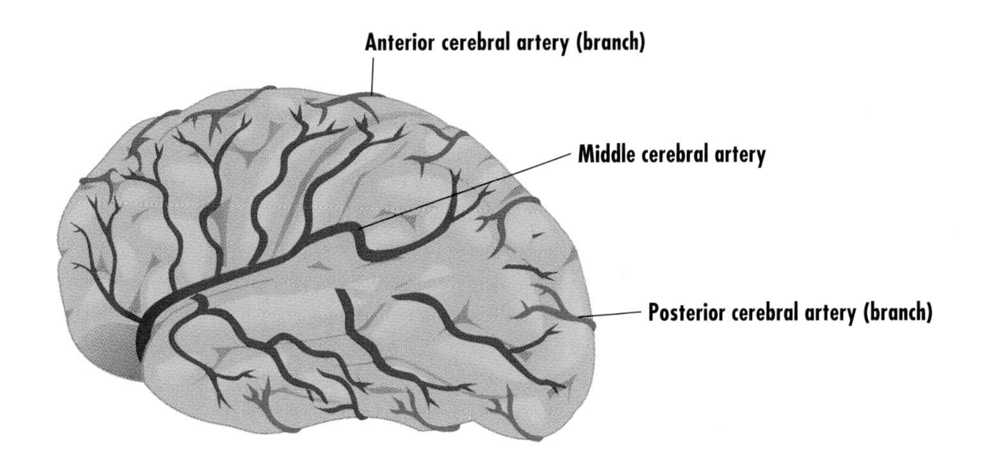

8 Migraine headaches may be caused by dilation (widening, distension) of the brain's arteries. Headache is also an important symptom of strokes caused by bleeding from an artery within the brain. In forms of stroke where a blood clot blocks the anterior or middle cerebral artery, headache may center in the forehead or temple.

Migraine

One common theory explaining migraine is presented here, but the field of migraine research is evolving, and new explanations may soon develop. Some new theories and new migraine therapies center around the neurotransmitter serotonin. Other theories suggest that migraine pain may be triggered by irritation of trigeminal nerve fibers that travel through the meninges.

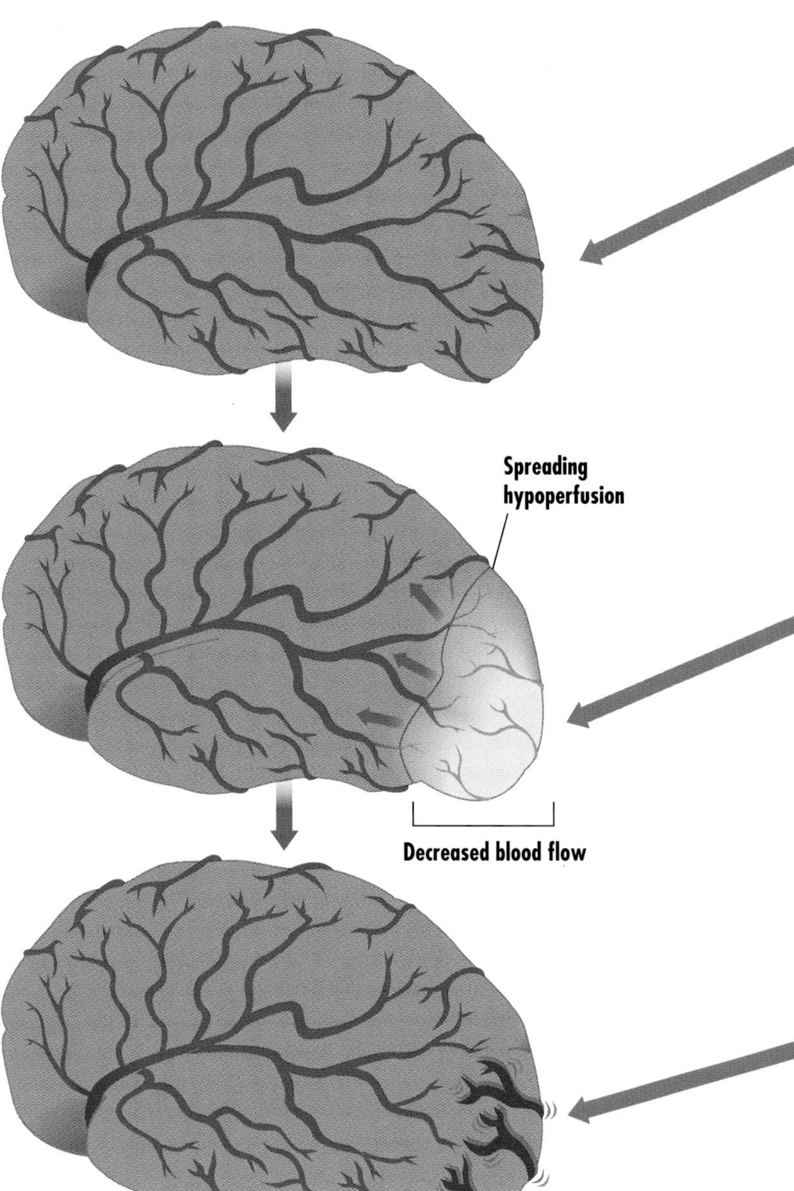

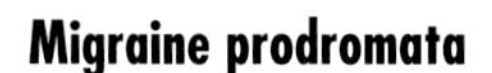

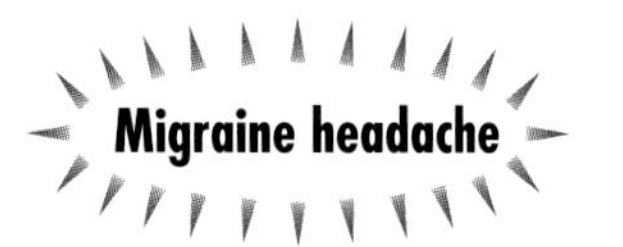

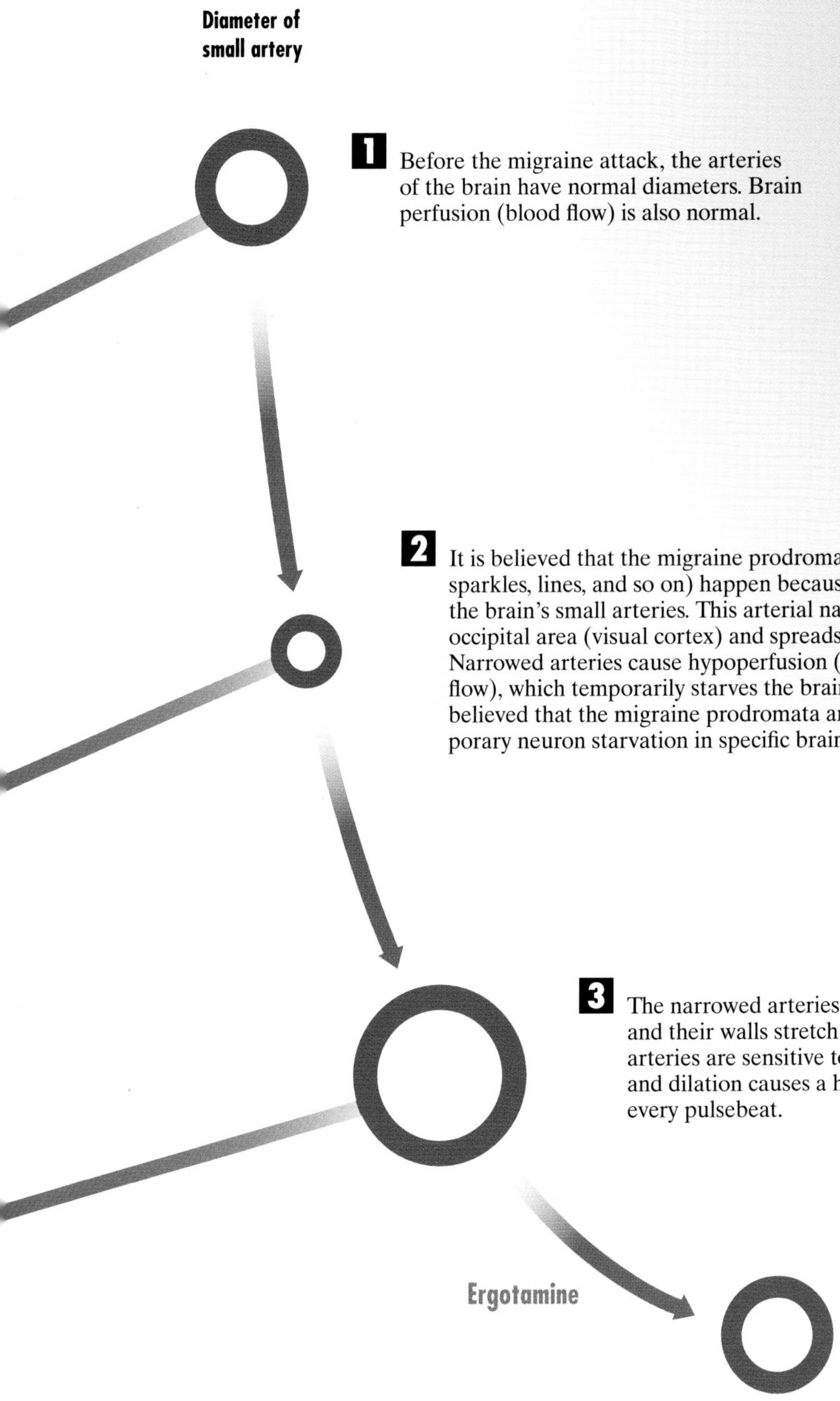

Diameter of small artery

1 Before the migraine attack, the arteries of the brain have normal diameters. Brain perfusion (blood flow) is also normal.

2 It is believed that the migraine prodromata (visual symptoms, sparkles, lines, and so on) happen because of constriction of the brain's small arteries. This arterial narrowing begins in the occipital area (visual cortex) and spreads forward in the brain. Narrowed arteries cause hypoperfusion (decreased blood flow), which temporarily starves the brain's local neurons. It is believed that the migraine prodromata are symptoms of temporary neuron starvation in specific brain areas.

3 The narrowed arteries suddenly widen (dilate), and their walls stretch out. Since the brain's arteries are sensitive to pain, their stretching and dilation causes a headache that throbs with every pulsebeat.

Ergotamine

4 Ergotamine constricts the widened arteries, returning them to a nearly normal diameter and stopping the headache pain. Some newer theories suggest that ergotamine also acts by blocking pain messages from nerves in the meninges. Sumatriptan, a newer migraine therapy, also constricts the brain's arteries and relieves migraine.

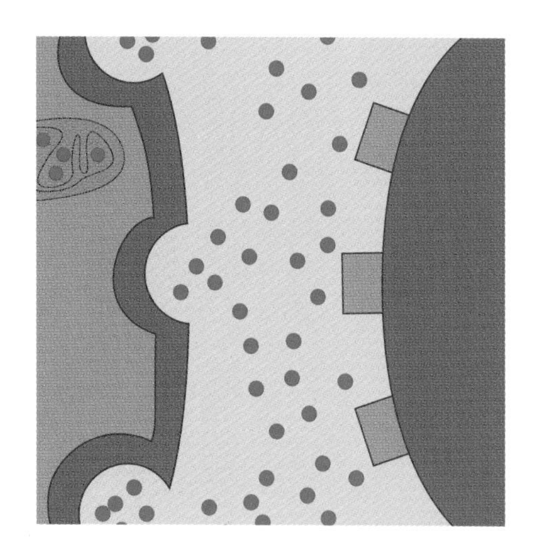

Psychiatric and Psychosomatic Illness

No Demons Here

BEFORE THE RISE of science in human history, humanity was ignorant and helpless before the forces of Nature. Superstition and fear clouded the way we looked at the natural world, and we explained the forces beyond our control as the work of demons, devils, and demigods. But now that we know the scientific explanations for the things that we feared, the demons and their counterparts have mostly disappeared. Those that have endured the longest may be the ones that we fear the most, the demons of mental illness.

Mental illness is as real a physical illness as diabetes, arthritis, or kidney disease. It affects as many as 48% of us in a lifetime and has many different forms. But the psychiatric symptoms of every form of mental illness, no matter how disturbing, are really only thoughts or actions that have somehow become disordered or painful. And because every human thought or action is the work of neurons, mental illness may be seen as neuron illness, or neuropsychiatric illness.

The exact causes of neuropsychiatric illness are unknown. The disease processes that underlie them are submicroscopic, so small that they remain undetectable by our best microscopes. Many scientists believe that mental illnesses are caused by an altered activity of neurotransmitters in specific areas of the brain. The symptoms of mental illness, abnormal thoughts or actions, are reflections of this altered neurotransmitter activity. While psychiatric medications probably act by correcting the neurotransmitter problem, psychotherapy and other forms of treatment are also helpful to many patients. It may be that the brain, like the heart and the limbs, recovers best when treated with a combination of therapies.

Neuropsychiatry is still in its infancy compared with other medical subspecialties, and psychiatrists know more about the pathology of some types of mental illness than others. Here we will examine only a few of the many forms of psychiatric illness, beginning with the two major disorders, schizophrenia and depression.

According to a series of studies done in the United States, between 0.6% and 1.9% of the population suffers from schizophrenia at some time in life. *Schizophrenia* usually attacks young people before age 40 and causes their mental functions to deteriorate. They often must leave their school or job. Some symptoms of schizophrenia include *delusions* (false, irrational beliefs) and *hallucinations* (false sensory perceptions).

In schizophrenia, thoughts and verbal communication are often disordered, causing looseness of associations or tangential thinking. *Looseness of associations* is the tendency to link unrelated ideas or to shift between subjects that are unrelated. *Tangential thinking* is the tendency to drift away from the subject of conversation or to give oblique or irrelevant answers to questions.

The symptoms of schizophrenia must last for six months or longer to help rule out other types of illness, including some types of metabolic disease. In many cases of schizophrenia, there is a family history of similar illness, leading to theories that the disease has an underlying genetic cause. It may be that one or more abnormal genes causes certain neurons in the brain to produce too much of the neurotransmitter dopamine. This theory is supported by the fact that the symptoms of schizophrenia can be relieved by drugs that block dopamine activity. These drugs include the phenothiazines (like thioridazine or fluphenazine) and haloperidol. Because these drugs block dopamine activity, they can also cause side effects similar to the symptoms of Parkinson's Disease (Chapter 5).

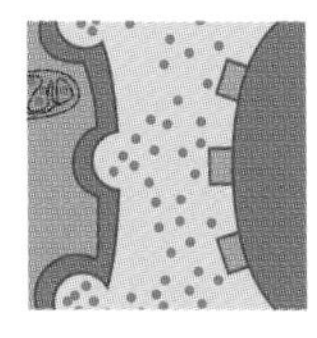

Depression is a form of mental illness characterized by excessive sadness. It is probably the most common form of psychiatric illness in the United States and may affect 10% of Americans annually. Depression often occurs together with a variety of other symptoms including the following: sleep disturbances, abrupt change in weight, poor concentration, feelings of worthlessness or guilt, fatigue (or sometimes restlessness), loss of interest in enjoyable activities, or recurrent thoughts of death or suicide. Some experts classify depression into two basic categories, exogenous depression and endogenous depression. In *exogenous depression*, the depressive symptoms appear after a painful or stressful life event, especially a loss of someone or something important. In *endogenous depression*, the symptoms seem to appear from within the psyche itself, without provocation.

Genetic factors appear to be important in endogenous depression. Studies in identical twins have shown that depression affects both twins in 75% of cases, and researchers have confirmed that depression generally runs in families.

Many theories have emerged about the neural mechanisms behind depression. Most have focused on complex imbalances in the activity of neurotransmitters within the brain, especially norepinephrine and serotonin.

Tricyclic antidepressant medications (TCAs), such as amitriptyline and imipramine, probably act by augmenting the effect of norepinephrine (and possibly serotonin) between neurons. TCAs block the mechanisms responsible for taking back this neurotransmitter into the neuron after it has been released at the synapse. When its recovery mechanism is blocked, norepinephrine lingers in the area of the synapse, and its activity between neurons is either intensified or prolonged. This appears to relieve depression.

Depression is also treated by drugs known as monoamine oxidase inhibitors, including phenelzine and tranylcypromine. These drugs inhibit monoamine oxidase (MAO), an enzyme system that degrades neurotransmitters that are monoamines, including norepinephrine. Inhibiting MAO stops the breakdown of norepinephrine and allows it to linger at the synapses. This prolongs or intensifies norepinephrine activity between neurons, and relieves depression.

Among the newest antidepressants are the serotonin reuptake inhibitors (SRIs), including fluoxetine and sertraline. These drugs appear to block systems that recover the neurotransmitter serotonin after it has been released. They relieve depression by intensifying or prolonging the activity of serotonin between neurons.

Anxiety can occur either alone or together with depression, schizophrenia, or many other illnesses. In its purest form, anxiety neurosis, it causes a feeling of dread or foreboding that may last for weeks or months.

Anxiety is often treated with one of the benzodiazepines, a family of medications that includes chlordiazepoxide, diazepam, and alprazolam. The benzodiazepines are used by 15% of Americans each year, and they are among the most widely prescribed drugs in the world. Benzodiazepines seem to enhance the activity of the neurotransmitter gamma-aminobutyric acid (GABA). GABA is a special type of neurotransmitter because it appears to reduce transmission of nerve impulses between neurons, which slows down certain types of brain activity.

Like mental illness, *psychosomatic illness* is often misunderstood. It is not imaginary; it is illness that reflects the mind's influence over other body organs. Just as the brain suffers when the heart or liver is ill, many body organs may suffer when the brain is stressed. Some researchers believe that people sometimes become sick when an upsetting environmental stress interacts with their own individual predisposition toward a certain medical illness. This predisposition may be inherited (genetic), secondary to injury (traumatic), or the result of a dangerous environment or personal habit (environmental). There is evidence for a psychosomatic component in many medical illnesses, although direct links have often been hard to prove. The actual mechanisms behind psychosomatic illness have been elusive as well.

Psychosomatic factors often affect the heart. Anxiety may account for the symptoms of 15% of patients who visit cardiologists, and psychosocial factors may account for up to 50% of a person's risk for coronary artery disease. Various forms of stress may engage the sympathetic branch of the autonomic nervous system, increasing heart rate and heart muscle contractility and increasing the heart's workload and demand for oxygen. When narrowed coronary arteries cannot meet the increased demands for blood (oxygen), the heart muscle may be starved for oxygen and send out pain signals in the form of angina.

In the lungs, anxiety has been known to trigger asthmatic attacks, and again the autonomic nervous system may be involved. Although the exact mechanism is unknown, there are theories that anxiety somehow signals the vagus nerve to contract muscles that narrow the breathing passages.

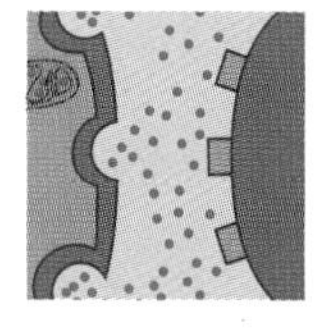

The digestive organs, because of their rich connections to the autonomic nervous system, are common sites of psychosomatic illnesses. About 25% of people with irritable bowel syndrome also have some type of psychiatric disorder, and their irritable bowel syndrome tends to be more severe. Both the onset and flare-up of Crohn's disease have also been linked to emotional distress. Peptic ulcer disease, which afflicts 12% of American men and 6% of women, has shown some response to antidepressants. Tricyclic antidepressants may help to heal ulcers, probably through a mechanism that decreases secretion of stomach acid.

Exciting new theories are evolving about brain-gut relationships in people with panic attacks who also suffer from certain bowel disorders. There is evidence that some of their intestinal distress may be orchestrated by the sympathetic nervous system, and possibly amplified through a nucleus of brain cells called the locus ceruleus, located in the pons.

Because the body also deals with stress by discharging glucocorticoids from the adrenal glands, the hypothalamus-pituitary-adrenal system is being studied for its possible relationship to psychosomatic illness. It is known that the adrenal glucocorticoid hormones (released as a response to stress through mechanisms that involve the brain and pituitary) can affect the metabolism of carbohydrates, fats, and proteins. They can also suppress the immune system and prevent inflammation. Recently, adrenal glucocorticoids have also been linked to depression through studies that show high levels of glucocorticoids in people whose depression followed a stressful life event (loss of spouse or job). Conversely, it is also known that many people who suffer from Cushing's disease (abnormally increased levels of adrenal glucocorticoids) often simultaneously suffer from depression. Added to this information has been the discovery that glucocorticoids can feed back to many areas of the brain, especially the limbic system's amygdala and hippocampus, and that glucocorticoids may influence the brain's secretion of neurotransmitters.

The result of all of this evidence is a theory that links stress-related secretion of glucocorticoids with glucocorticoid effects on many different body organs (possibly triggering psychosomatic illnesses), through a mechanism that activates and feeds back to areas of the brain that regulate emotion and memory. In sum, it may be that stress is linked to both depression and psychosomatic illness though the glucocorticoid stress hormones of the adrenal glands.

It's easy to see, then, how psychosomatic factors could possibly contribute to the cause or course of many different illnesses. Other illnesses currently being studied for a psychosomatic relationship include cancer, ulcerative colitis, adult-onset diabetes, and rheumatoid arthritis.

Psychiatric Illness: Where and Why

1 Schizophrenia has been linked to overactivity of the neurotransmitter dopamine. Here are some important pathways in the brain where dopamine is used as a neurotransmitter in synapses. Dopamine activity is heavy in the frontal lobes and amygdala, which may help explain why thought disorders are seen in schizophrenia.

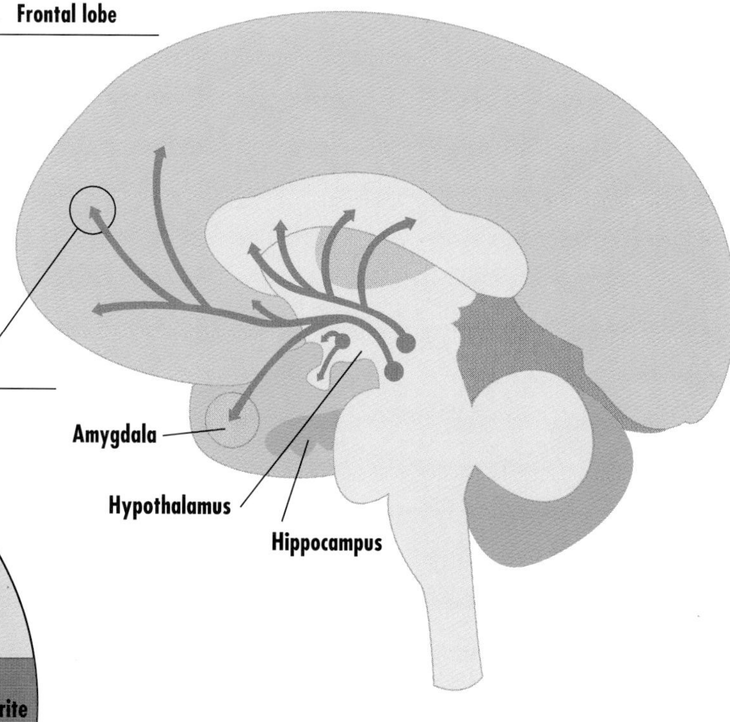

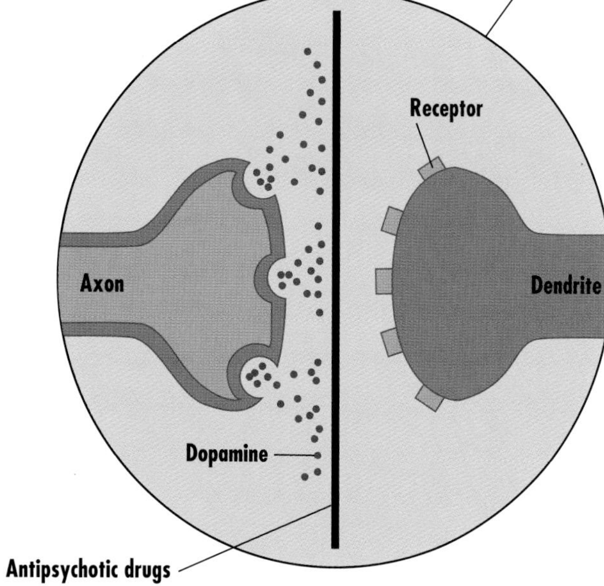

2 Schizophrenia is treated with antipsychotic drugs, including the phenothiazines and haloperidol. These medicines act by blocking the activity of the neurotransmitter dopamine at synapses in the brain. The exact mechanism is unknown.

4 Normally, extra norepinephrine within the neuron is broken down by the monoamine oxidase (MAO) enzyme system inside tiny cellular organs called mitochondria.

5 The MAO inhibitors block the MAO enzyme system. This stops the breakdown of norepinephrine, increases norepinephrine activity at the synapses, and relieves depression.

3 Depression has been linked to the decreased activity of the neurotransmitters norepinephrine and serotonin in the brain. Some major pathways that use norepinephrine (blue) and serotonin (pink) are shown here. The pathways indicate heavy activity in parts of the limbic system and may explain why depression affects emotion, appetite, and thought processing. Medications that relieve depression work by increasing the activity of either norepinephrine or serotonin at synapses in the brain.

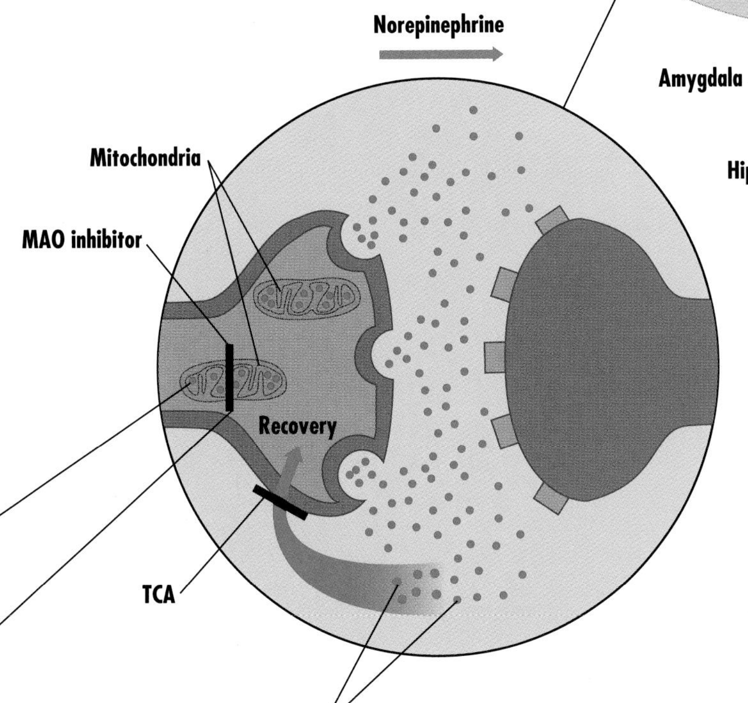

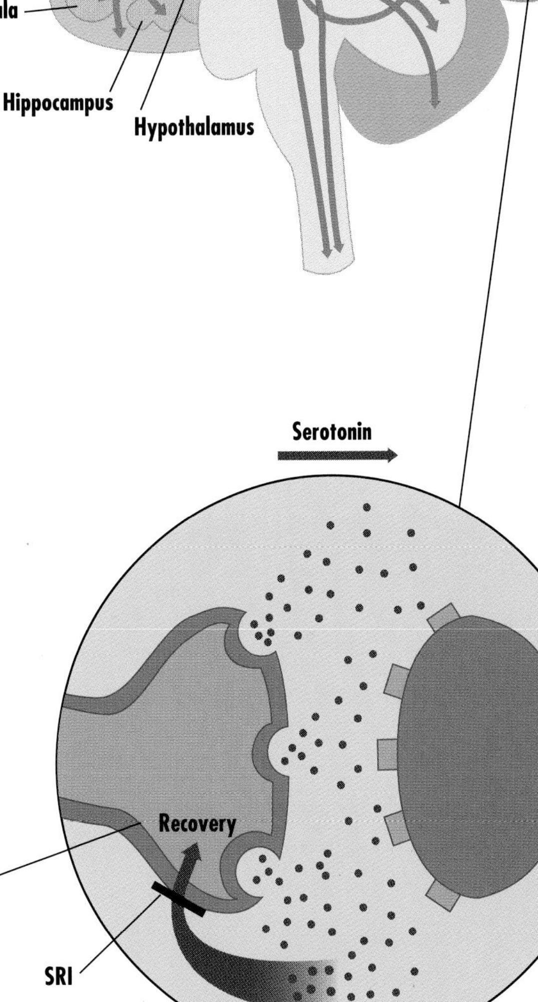

6 Normally, extra norepinephrine at the synapse is taken back into the neuron by a recovery system. Tricyclic antidepressants (TCAs) block the recovery system and allow more norepinephrine to remain outside the neuron. This increases norepinephrine activity at the synapse and relieves depression.

7 Normally, extra serotonin at the synapse is also taken back into the neuron by its own recovery system. The serotonin reuptake inhibitors (SRIs), such as fluoxetine and sertraline, block this recovery system. This allows more serotonin to remain within the synapse and relieves depression.

Mind and Body: New Frontiers

1 Stress can engage both the body's adrenal glucocorticoid hormones and parts of the autonomic nervous system (especially the sympathetic nervous system). Theories about how emotional or psychic stress may cause or exacerbate illness have focused on both these areas. Stress may engage the adrenal glucocorticoids through pathways (shown here as blue arrows) that involve the limbic system, hypothalamus, and pituitary. The pituitary, at the command of the hypothalamus, secretes ACTH, which stimulates the adrenals to produce adrenal glucocorticoids (its stress hormones).

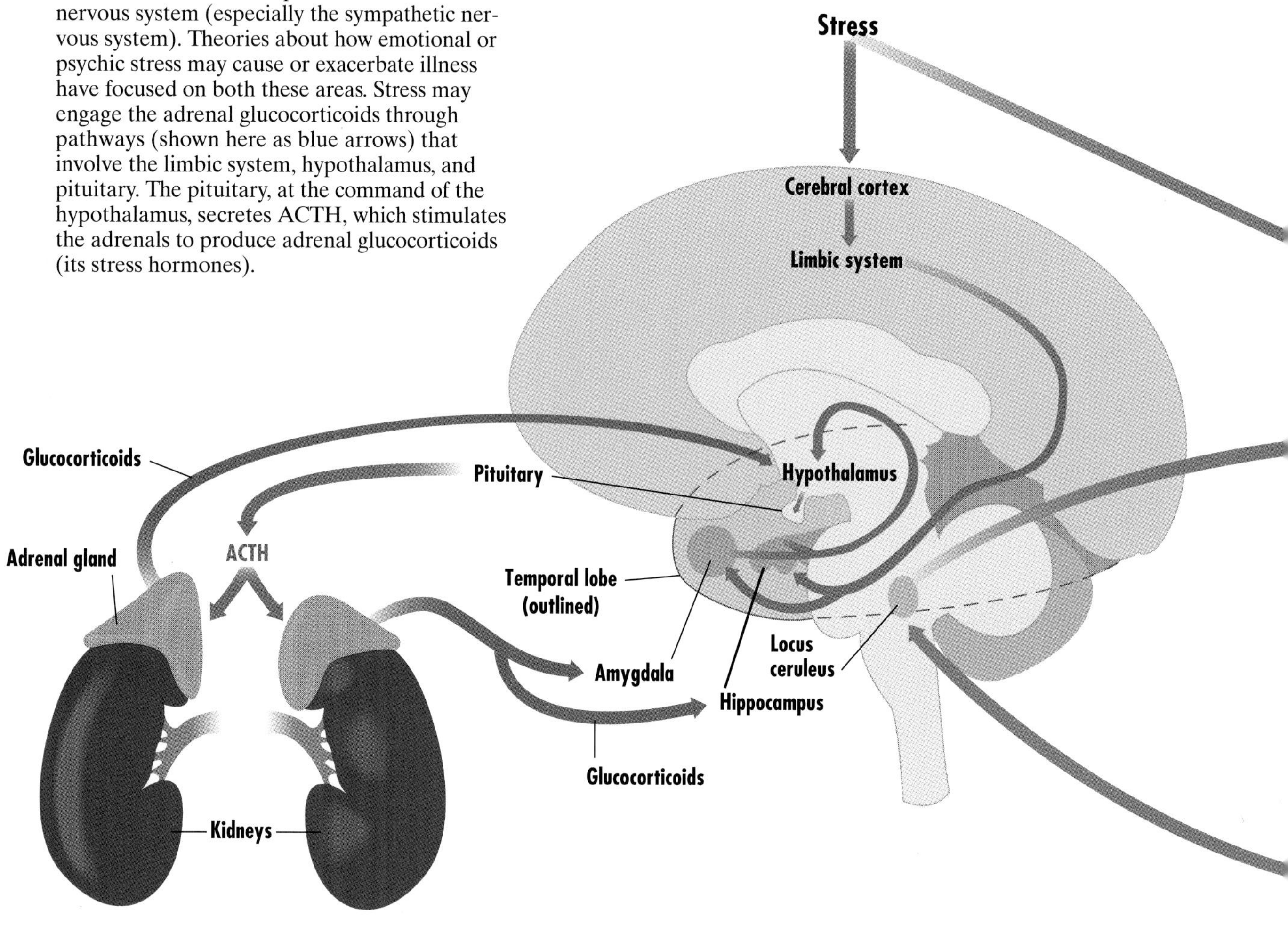

2 Adrenal glucocorticoids have widespread effects on many body systems, including metabolism, inflammatory responses, and immunity from disease. They also feed back (red arrows) to many brain areas, including limbic areas linked to emotion and memory. It is possible that stress causes both psychosomatic illness and depression by way of adrenal glucocorticoid stress hormones.

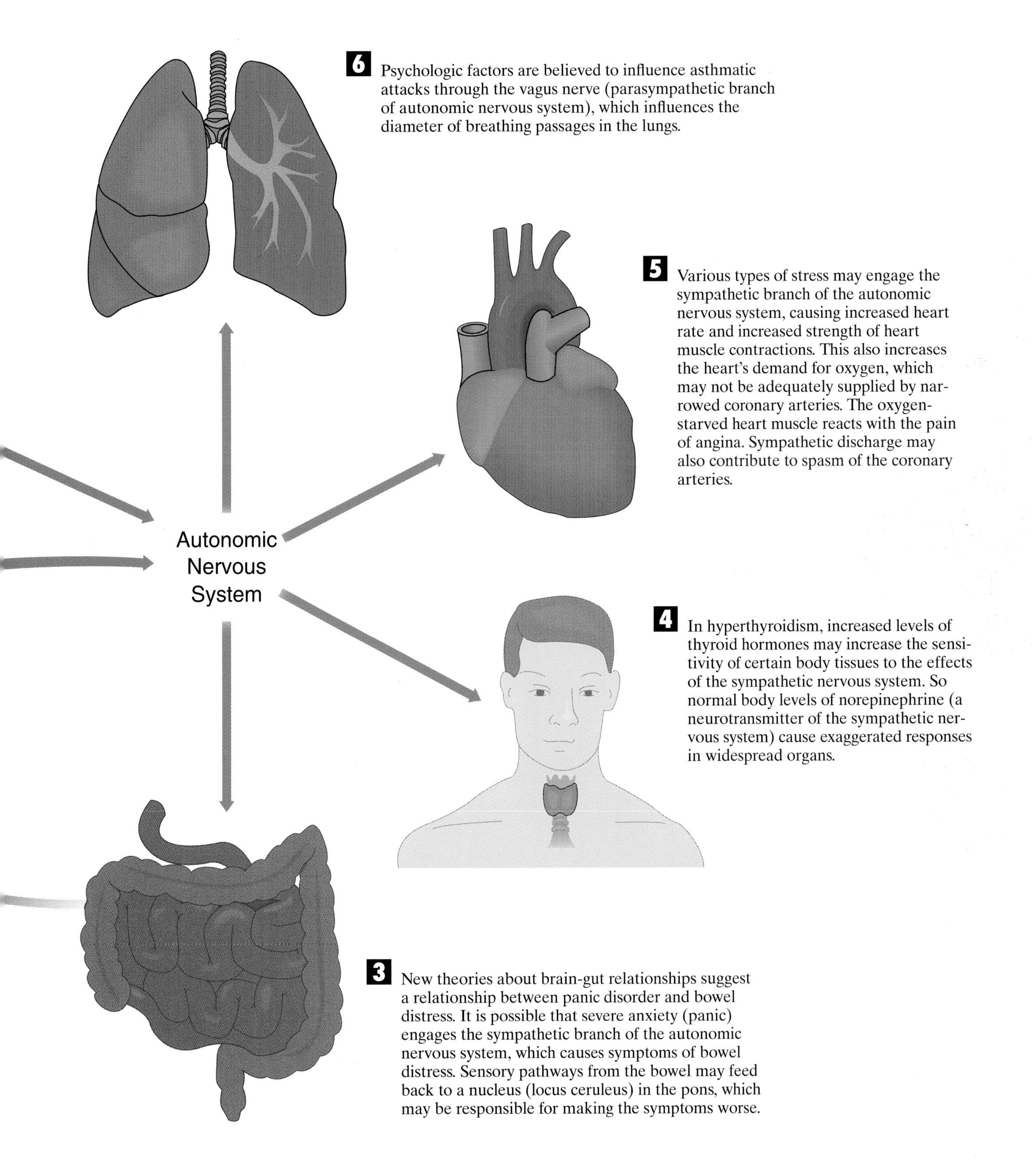

6 Psychologic factors are believed to influence asthmatic attacks through the vagus nerve (parasympathetic branch of autonomic nervous system), which influences the diameter of breathing passages in the lungs.

5 Various types of stress may engage the sympathetic branch of the autonomic nervous system, causing increased heart rate and increased strength of heart muscle contractions. This also increases the heart's demand for oxygen, which may not be adequately supplied by narrowed coronary arteries. The oxygen-starved heart muscle reacts with the pain of angina. Sympathetic discharge may also contribute to spasm of the coronary arteries.

4 In hyperthyroidism, increased levels of thyroid hormones may increase the sensitivity of certain body tissues to the effects of the sympathetic nervous system. So normal body levels of norepinephrine (a neurotransmitter of the sympathetic nervous system) cause exaggerated responses in widespread organs.

3 New theories about brain-gut relationships suggest a relationship between panic disorder and bowel distress. It is possible that severe anxiety (panic) engages the sympathetic branch of the autonomic nervous system, which causes symptoms of bowel distress. Sensory pathways from the bowel may feed back to a nucleus (locus ceruleus) in the pons, which may be responsible for making the symptoms worse.

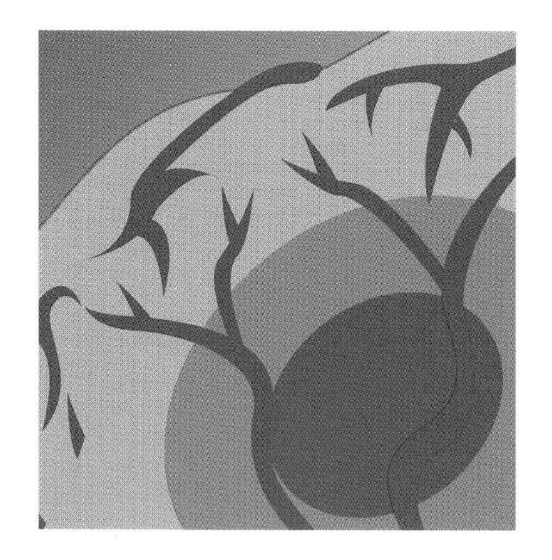

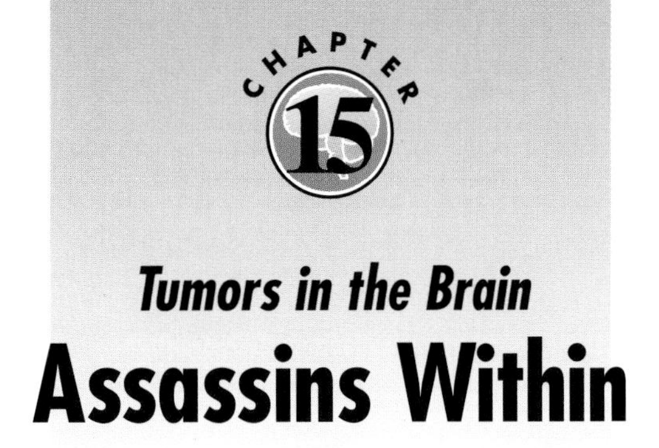

Tumors in the Brain

Assassins Within

EVERY SOCIETY FEARS the enemy who strikes from within, either the outsider who infiltrates the native population or the native who turns on his brothers and sisters. In human societies, we call these assassins "terrorists" and "traitors"; in the brain we call them tumors. Tumors of the brain and spinal cord kill 90,000 Americans annually and account for 25% of all U.S. healthcare dollars spent on cancer treatment.

When a brain tumor is small and slow growing, the brain may compensate well and show no symptoms, but when a tumor reaches about 3 centimeters (about 1¼ inch) in size, it begins to compress the brain. The brain's blood supply and the circulation of cerebrospinal fluid are also disrupted, and the blood-brain barrier in the area around the tumor is weakened. Small blood vessels begin to leak proteins and water, causing the brain to swell, a condition called vasogenic cerebral edema. The tumor infiltrates and displaces normal brain structures, causing neurologic symptoms that vary depending on tumor location. As the tumor grows, there may be cell death (necrosis) or bleeding (hemorrhage) inside it.

Symptoms. Headaches, characteristically occurring in the middle of the night or in the morning when the patient awakens, are the first symptom in 50% of people with brain tumors. The headache pain may be due to tumor toxins that irritate the pain-sensitive structures within the skull (Chapter 13) or to tumor traction on dura or blood vessels. Headaches vary in their severity and quality and sometimes feel more like a vague discomfort rather than real pain. Frontal and temporal tumors often cause headaches in the frontal or temporal areas of the head or in back of the eyes, while tumors of the cerebellum and lower parts of the brain often cause headaches in the occipital area or in back of the ears.

The onset of seizures is the first symptom of 20% of patients with brain tumors. Seizures may be triggered when tumor toxins and chemicals leaked from damaged cells irritate neurons and cause them to fire abnormally. In fast-growing tumors, the seizures tend to be focal (partial) seizures, whose symptoms (sensory, motor, and so on) are related to the tumor's location in the brain. So a frontal tumor gives motor seizures, while an occipital tumor generates seizures with visual abnormalities. In slow-growing tumors, seizures are more often generalized. Sometimes a patient may suffer from seizures for months or years before the underlying brain tumor is discovered.

Brain tumors may also cause gastrointestinal symptoms, including poor appetite, nausea followed by vomiting, or vomiting that is not preceded by nausea. Gastrointestinal symptoms are more common in children, and in adults whose tumors are located in the cerebellum or lower parts of the brain.

People with brain tumors often experience changes in neural function. As the tumor grows, its associated destruction and brain edema may cause either a general decline in mental abilities or a specific series of mental changes that reflect the tumor's location in the brain. Tumors in the temporal lobes, for example, may cause auditory hallucinations (because of auditory cortex involvement), mood shifts, or changes in personality that mimic psychiatric problems. Occipital or parietal tumors can cause loss of vision (visual cortex involvement), spatial disorientation, and problems in communication. Frontal tumors, which can grow to be very large before they affect mental abilities, tend to cause symptoms that are vague and difficult to pinpoint. With frontal tumors, thoughts and actions may become less spontaneous, performance at work may not be as "sharp" as before, and apathy and lethargy may gradually overshadow the patient's life. In every location the presence of tumor, with its leaking toxins and spreading destruction, changes the normal environment around neurons and either causes them to fire abnormally or injures them so they cannot fire at all. Tumors can also kill neurons directly, either by manufacturing toxins or by competing with neurons for life-giving food and oxygen from nearby blood vessels.

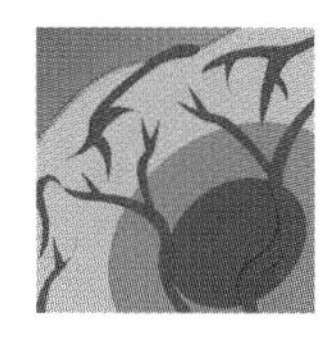

Sometimes the combination of large tumor size and brain edema (swelling) causes dangerous shifts in the normal position of the brain around the tumor. The expanding tumor compresses neighboring parts of the brain and pushes them under natural folds of the dura or down into the foramen magnum. This is called herniation. Herniation of parts of the brain can cause compression of important cerebral arteries, cerebrospinal fluid pathways, and cranial nerves. Herniation of the brain downward into the foramen magnum can compress parts of the medulla that regulate vital functions (such as the respiratory centers). This can cause the patient to stop breathing. Since herniations of the brain can be life-threatening emergencies, they are treated immediately with intravenous medications that reduce brain swelling. Sometimes emergency procedures to remove fluid are also needed.

Although the symptoms discussed here are common to all brain tumors regardless of origin, they are more likely to develop rapidly (over a period of days or weeks) in patients who have a metastatic tumor rather than a primary tumor of the brain.

Metastatic tumors. In adults, most tumors that affect the brain come from outside the brain's own population. They are *metastases*, tumors that have spread—metastasized—from primary cancers arising in other parts of the body. During the course of their illnesses, 25% to 35% of all cancer patients will see their cancers metastasize to the brain: 50%

to 65% of melanomas, 40% to 60% of lung cancers, and 20% to 51% of breast cancers. Cancers of the colon and rectum, sarcomas, kidney cancer, and ovarian cancer may attack the brain as well. Lung cancer and melanomas often cause metastatic tumors at multiple sites in the brain, while cancers of the kidney, lung, and breast are more likely to cause only a single brain metastasis. In more than 80% of cancer patients, brain metastases are discovered after their primary cancer has already been diagnosed, but in the remaining 20% the symptoms of brain involvement lead to discovery of a primary cancer elsewhere in the body.

Most tumors metastasize to the brain in a step-by-step pattern through the bloodstream. Small clumps of tumor cells first enter the circulation at the site of primary cancer and initially metastasize to the lungs, liver, or lymph nodes. From metastases in these organs, tumor cells enter the bloodstream again and metastasize to the brain. In some studies, the average time between diagnosis of a primary cancer elsewhere and subsequent diagnosis of a brain metastasis was found to be about 17 months. Lung cancer, renal cancer, and melanoma tend to spread to the brain quickly, while sarcomas, breast cancer, and colon cancer spread more slowly.

Either radiation alone, or radiation after surgical treatment, is used to treat metastatic cancer in the brain. Steroids are prescribed to relieve brain edema because they stablize cell membranes and decrease inflammation. They are especially effective in relieving generalized symptoms, such as headache and confusion, which tend to reflect the amount of brain swelling inside the skull. Osmotherapy, using medicines that draw excess water from areas of brain edema, is also helpful.

Primary brain tumors. When a tumor arises from the brain's own population, it is called a primary brain tumor. Primary brain tumors usually come not from groups of renegade neurons, but from one of the many populations of neuroglia. Tumors that arise from neuroglia are called gliomas.

In adults, 75% of gliomas are malignant astrocytomas (also called glioblastoma or malignant glioma). They generally strike middle-aged adults and are very difficult to treat. If the tumor is in an area of the brain that is accessible to surgery, as much as possible of the tumor is removed before the patient is given radiation treatments and chemotherapy.

Primary brain tumors are the second most common cause of cancer death in children under age 15. Most of the primary brain tumors of childhood also arise from the neuroglia.

About 40% of childhood brain tumors affect the cerebellum, which is the single most common site for brain tumors in children. Most of these cerebellar tumors are astrocytomas. They are removed surgically, resulting in a high long-term survival rate.

Tumors of the Brain: Enemies, Foreign and Domestic

1 In adults, most tumors that affect the brain are metastases, or metastatic tumors. These are cancers that have spread to the brain from primary sites in other body organs. Melanoma, the potentially deadly skin cancer, and cancers of the lung and breast commonly spread to the brain by passing in a step-by-step pattern through the bloodstream. Melanoma often kills by spreading to the brain. Here we follow the path of a metastatic melanoma that has invaded through the skin and has begun to metastasize.

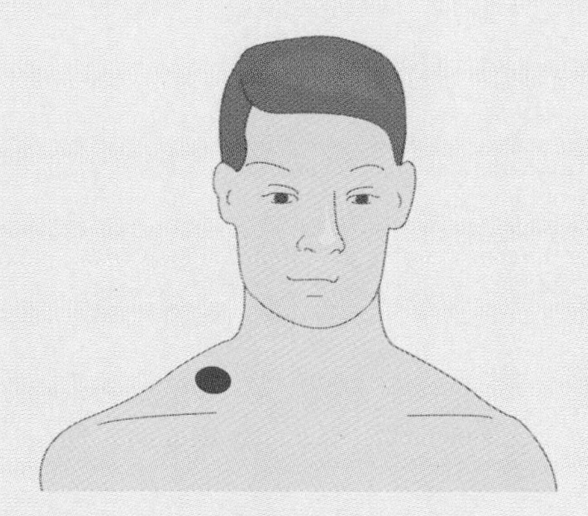

2 Clumps of melanoma tumor cells pass into the bloodstream near their primary site in the skin. They travel to the lungs or liver and begin to grow there as sites of metastatic melanoma.

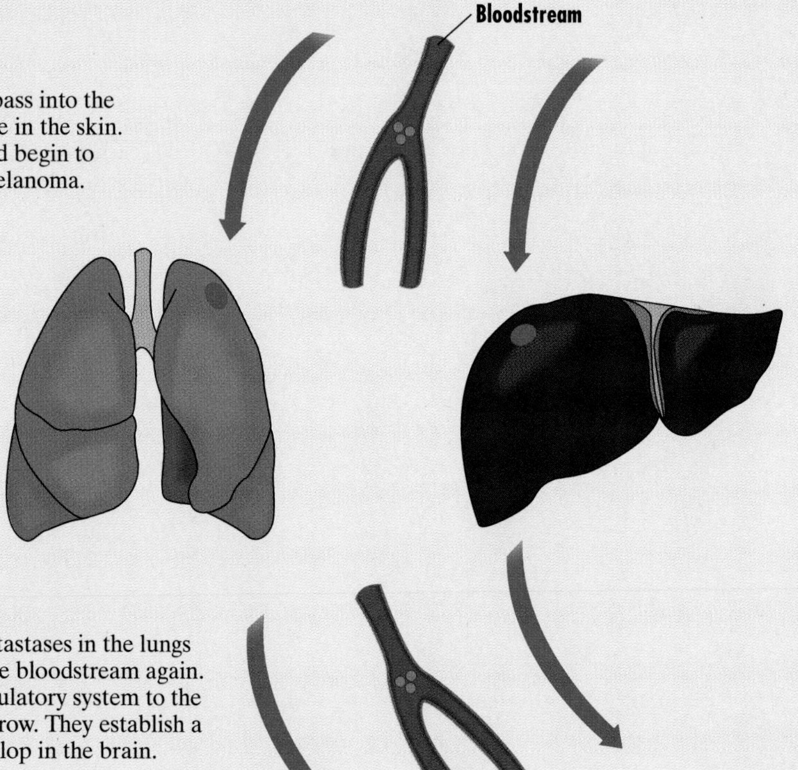

3 From sites of melanoma metastases in the lungs or liver, tumor cells enter the bloodstream again. They travel through the circulatory system to the brain, where they begin to grow. They establish a site for a skin tumor to develop in the brain.

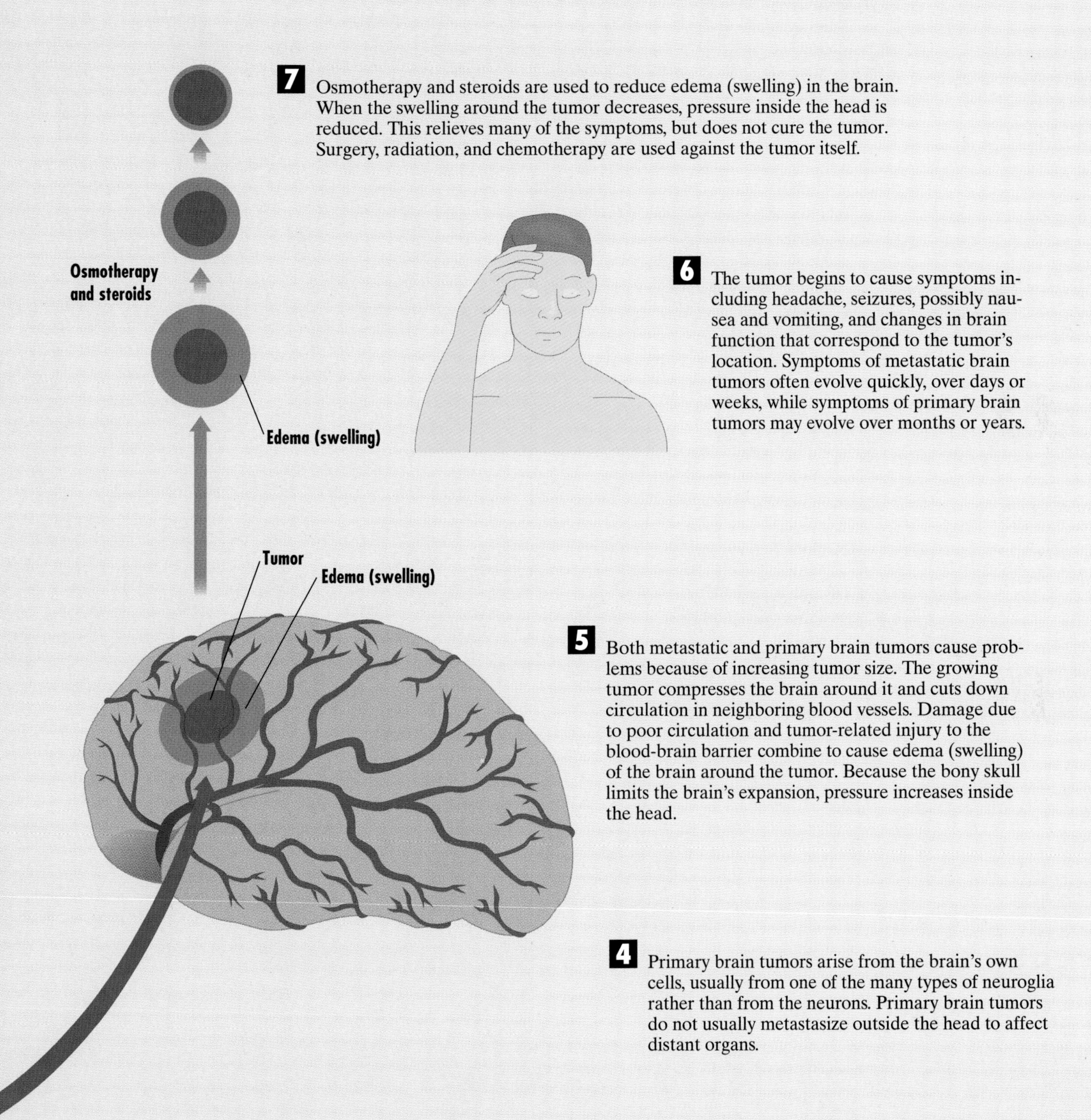

7 Osmotherapy and steroids are used to reduce edema (swelling) in the brain. When the swelling around the tumor decreases, pressure inside the head is reduced. This relieves many of the symptoms, but does not cure the tumor. Surgery, radiation, and chemotherapy are used against the tumor itself.

6 The tumor begins to cause symptoms including headache, seizures, possibly nausea and vomiting, and changes in brain function that correspond to the tumor's location. Symptoms of metastatic brain tumors often evolve quickly, over days or weeks, while symptoms of primary brain tumors may evolve over months or years.

5 Both metastatic and primary brain tumors cause problems because of increasing tumor size. The growing tumor compresses the brain around it and cuts down circulation in neighboring blood vessels. Damage due to poor circulation and tumor-related injury to the blood-brain barrier combine to cause edema (swelling) of the brain around the tumor. Because the bony skull limits the brain's expansion, pressure increases inside the head.

4 Primary brain tumors arise from the brain's own cells, usually from one of the many types of neuroglia rather than from the neurons. Primary brain tumors do not usually metastasize outside the head to affect distant organs.

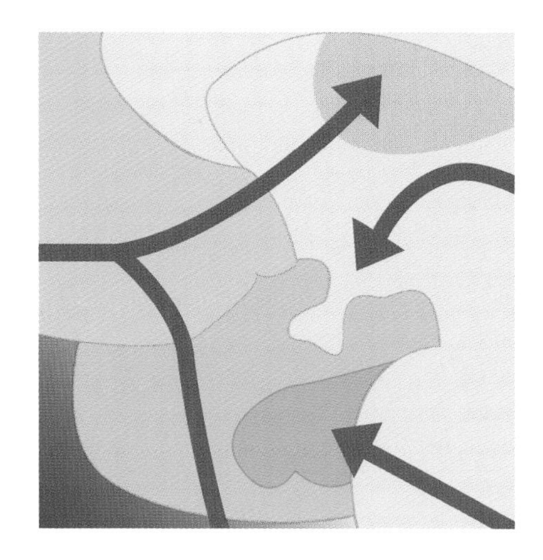

Toxins and the Brain

Environmental Disasters

THE MORE WE study the Earth's environment, the more we appreciate the fragile balance that underlies the function of our natural world. Humankind's most recent history—the last 10 to 15 decades—has seen us damage our Earth's environment in many ways. We have done harm out of ignorance and out of denial. And sometimes, even with clear knowledge of the consequences, we have done harm by choice.

Some of us deal with our brains in the same way.

In the neural world, each individual neuron fills a distinct niche in the complex ecology of the brain, and each individual neuron, because it can be neither reproduced nor replaced, becomes an extinct species when it dies. Neurons may be damaged or killed by a wide range of toxic substances. Volumes of information have been written about the various types of substance abuse and about their implications for the individual and for society. Here we will simply examine how various chemicals interfere with "how your brain works." Their destructive impact on the beauty of the neural world, like the burning of a rain forest or the devastation caused by an oil spill, will speak for itself.

Alcohol. About 70% of Americans use alcohol on occasion, and about 12% of these are "heavy drinkers" who consume alcohol daily and become intoxicated several times a month. Neural damage caused by alcohol alone is often difficult to assess because of the presence of other toxic substances, called congeners, that occur together with alcohol in different alcoholic beverages, giving them their characteristic colors and flavors. Congeners include methanol, butanol, aldehydes, esters, histamine, and sometimes iron, lead, or cobalt.

In general, after causing some brief initial feelings of stimulation and euphoria, alcohol acts as a depressant by decreasing the activity of neurons. Although the exact mechanism is unknown, alcohol seems to affect several different types of neurotransmitters simultaneously and changes certain fluid characteristics within the neuron membranes. Neurons that are chronically exposed to alcohol seem to adjust either their cell membranes or their internal chemical reactions to compensate for the presence of alcohol. Eventually, they adapt to function best in an alcohol-rich environment and actually come to *require* alcohol to perform optimally. This is the basis for physical addiction, and it is the reason that alcoholics suffer withdrawal symptoms when they stop drinking.

Acute alcohol ingestion can cause a wide range of symptoms, including irregular behavior, slurred speech, lack of coordination, abnormal gait, inattention, drowsiness, and coma. Large amounts of alcohol (generally between three and five times what is required for legal "intoxication") can cause death by depressing areas in the medulla that control breathing.

Chronic use of alcohol has been linked to enlargement of the brain's ventricles, widening of its sulci, and possibly atrophy (shrinking) of the cerebral cortex. Along with these changes comes a decrease in certain cortical functions, including motor performance and short-term memory. Abstinence tends to reverse many of these changes after a year or more without alcohol, although some memory problems may remain, possibly because of damage to areas below the cortex.

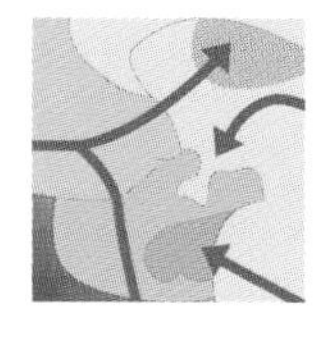

If alcoholic beverages are consumed in place of a normal diet, there may be many severe vitamin and mineral deficiencies. For example, Wernicke-Korsakoff syndrome, which is caused by thiamine deficiency, is a common disease of the alcoholic population living in the large cities of Western countries. In Wernicke-Korsakoff syndrome, neurons and their nerve fibers are damaged in the thalamus, hypothalamus, cerebellar vermis, and elsewhere. Symptoms include confusion, disorientation, amnesia, and difficulties in walking and eye movement.

"Alcoholic" cerebellar degeneration occurs in people who have a history of prolonged heavy use of alcohol. In this disease all types of brain cells degenerate in the vermis and upper portions of the cortex of the cerebellum. Purkinje cells are particularly affected. The symptoms include instability of the trunk of the body and a wide-based (and hence more stable) stance and gait. Good nutrition stops progression of the disease and may improve symptoms.

Heavy chronic alcohol use seems to have toxic effects on the limbic system and on hypothalamic control of the pituitary. Symptoms include problems in sexual desire and sexual functioning, reduction of menstrual periods in women, and even infertility. In about 50% of male alcoholics, increased levels of female hormones can cause breast enlargement and a female pattern of hair distribution around the area of the genitalia.

Chronic alcohol exposure in pregnant women may cause problems in the developing fetus, and children born to severely alcoholic mothers may suffer from fetal alcohol syndrome, with its characteristic low birth weight, slight microcephaly, and heart abnormalities. As infants, such children may be irritable and have problems feeding and sleeping. In school, they may have problems learning. The exact mechanism behind fetal alcohol syndrome is not known. The cause may be alcohol alone or a combination of factors including toxic effects of the by-products of alcohol breakdown, smoking, and poor nutrition in the mother.

When chronic use of alcohol is abruptly stopped, neurons that have adjusted to the alcohol-rich environment suddenly find themselves free of the inhibiting effects of this drug. They become uninhibited and overactive, and this reaction underlies many of the symptoms of alcohol withdrawal. These symptoms include shakes or jitters, dysfunction of the autonomic nervous system (rapid heartbeat and breathing, elevated body temperature), anxiety or panic attacks, and problems sleeping. Shakes or jitters usually begin first, within 5–10 hours after the last dose of alcohol. Symptoms peak on day 2 or 3 and are usually improved by day 4 or 5. In about 5% of alcoholics the symptoms progress to become delirium tremens (DTs), where withdrawal is associated with confusion, delusions, hallucinations, and sometimes generalized seizures.

In general, people who suffer from alcoholism, and who remain untreated, can expect to shorten their life span by about 15 years.

Opioids. The opioids are a group of related substances that bind to opioid receptors in many areas of the body. Some opioids occur naturally in poppy juice, some are semisynthetic, and some are entirely synthetic. Included in the opiates are morphine, codeine, diacetylmorphine (heroin), hydromorphone, meperidine, and others.

When opioids bind to opioid receptors they have varying effects that correlate with the area of the brain involved. Their binding to receptors in the medulla causes nausea and vomiting; in the spinal cord and thalamus they cause decreased perception of pain; in the limbic system they cause euphoria; and in the reticular activating system they cause sedation. Opioids depress normal breathing activity by decreasing the brain's response to higher levels of carbon dioxide in the blood. In the area of the hypothalamus and pituitary, opioids decrease secretion of hormones, specifically LH (leading to a decrease in testosterone) and thyrotropin, but they increase prolactin.

Overdose of opioids causes unresponsiveness, respiratory depression (only 2 to 4 breaths per minute), decreased heart rate and body temperature, and constricted pupils. If not treated, opioid overdose can cause death from respiratory depression and cardiorespiratory arrest (the heart and lungs stop working). Opioid overdose is treated with naloxone.

Statistics show that people who persistently use opiates have an increased risk of death from suicide, homicide, accidents, and infections (especially AIDS, tuberculosis, and hepatitis).

Cocaine and Amphetaminelike substances. Cocaine comes from the leaves of the coca plant. It is a stimulant and a local anesthetic, and it causes blood vessels to constrict. Cocaine affects neurons that use the neurotransmitters dopamine, norepinephrine, and serotonin. It causes changes in the cell membranes of neurons, and these changes prevent the re-uptake of neurotransmitters after they have been released into synapses.

Like cocaine, the amphetamines block the re-uptake of dopamine, and possibly also the re-uptake of norepinephrine and serotonin. By some unknown mechanism, amphetamines also seem to enhance dopamine release.

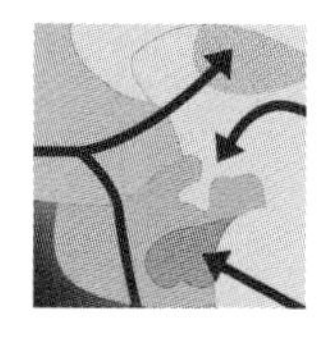

Cocaine and the amphetamines act at many levels of the brain, wherever there are synapses that use the neurotransmitters whose re-uptake they affect. They cause feelings of euphoria, increased alertness, decreased hunger, and decreased need for sleep. They may also cause feelings of paranoia and suspicion that mimic symptoms of psychiatric illness, particularly paranoid schizophrenia. Hallucinations, especially of bugs or vermin crawling under the skin, have also been described.

High doses of cocaine can cause irregular heartbeat and spasms of the coronary arteries that lead to a heart attack (myocardial infarction). Cocaine may also increase blood pressure to the point of causing brain hemorrhage.

Withdrawal from cocaine or amphetamines is associated with feelings of unhappiness and depression, agitation and fatigue. There may be feelings of sleepiness (but an inability to sleep), and there is often a craving for food.

Marijuana. A family of chemical compounds called cannabinoids is found in the marijuana plant. The cannabinoids' mechanism of action is unknown, and no cannabinoid receptors have yet been found. Studies in primates have suggested that marijuana affects memory by decreasing the activity of neurons in the hippocampus. It may also block the hypothalamic releasing hormone that regulates secretion of FSH and LH (which, in turn, regulate secretion of sex hormones). In men, marijuana can decrease the quality and quantity of sperm, an effect that is probably reversible when marijuana use is stopped.

Acutely, marijuana causes dry mouth and rapid heartbeat, elevates mood, and gives the sensation that time is passing more slowly. It also impairs performance on complex tasks, such as driving a car. People who use marijuana may become passive, apathetic, and sleepy, or sometimes anxious and paranoid. Use of marijuana may also trigger a relapse in people who have a history of schizophrenia.

Some experts suggest that chronic use of marijuana causes an "amotivational syndrome," whose symptoms include reduced drive, lethargy, mild depression, and loss of interest in activities that were once enjoyed.

Why Addiction? There is increasing evidence that alcoholism is not a moral weakness but a biologically influenced disorder. Children of alcoholics seem to have a fourfold increased risk of developing alcoholism themselves, even if they are adopted by nonalcoholic parents. Even before alcoholism develops, some children of alcoholics appear to become less intoxicated at a given blood level of alcohol than those not at risk for alcoholism. They may have inherited a nervous system that is less sensitive to the intoxicating effects of alcohol.

So far there is no consistent evidence for a biologic basis in opioid addiction, although some people addicted to opioids have alcoholic or drug-dependent parents. Studies have shown that many people with opioid dependence have coexisting psychiatric disorders (depression, anxiety, antisocial personality), but the relationship to opioid use is unknown.

Although it has been suggested that some people turn to cocaine for relief of preexisting psychiatric disorders, many people who abuse cocaine do not have preexisting psychiatric problems.

Alcohol: Pollution at Multiple Sites

1 Alcohol, also called ethanol, causes both acute and chronic problems. It has direct effects on the brain and secondary effects due to alcohol-induced damage to other organs. Alcohol-induced damage may be complicated by the additional toxic effects of congeners—chemicals that occur together with alcohol in alcoholic beverages.

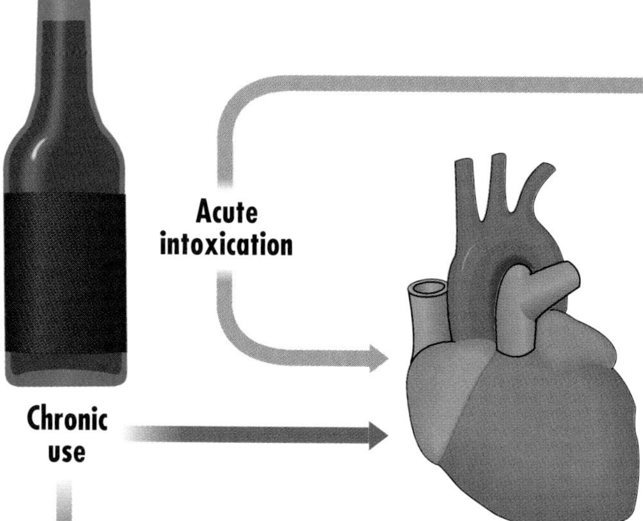

3 Acutely, an alcohol binge can trigger "holiday heart" syndrome, a rapid irregular heartbeat (atrial or ventricular arrhythmia). Chronic heavy drinking can contribute to high blood pressure, damage heart muscle, and impair heart function. In alcoholics, periods of heavy drinking have been associated with strokes.

4 Pregnant women who are chronic heavy drinkers can give birth to children suffering from fetal alcohol syndrome. These infants may have abnormally low birth weight, microcephaly, heart problems, and learning difficulties. Smoking and poor nutrition in pregnant alcoholics may compound alcohol's effects on the fetus.

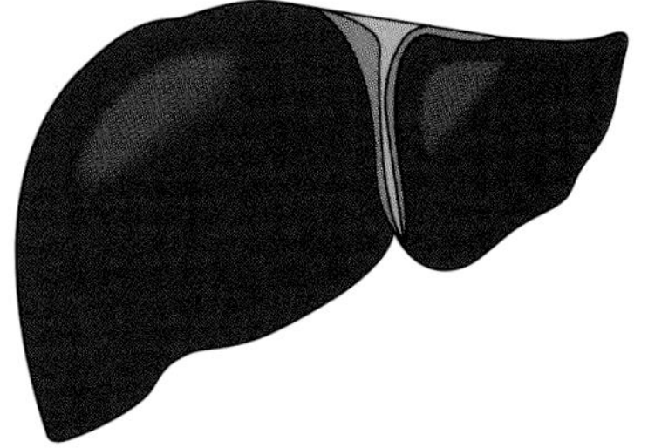

5 Chronic heavy alcohol use can harm the brain indirectly by causing liver damage (alcoholic hepatitis and cirrhosis). Eventually, the damaged liver loses its normal ability to remove toxins from the blood. Toxins (especially ammonia) accumulate and damage the brain, causing confusion, drowsiness, stupor, or coma.

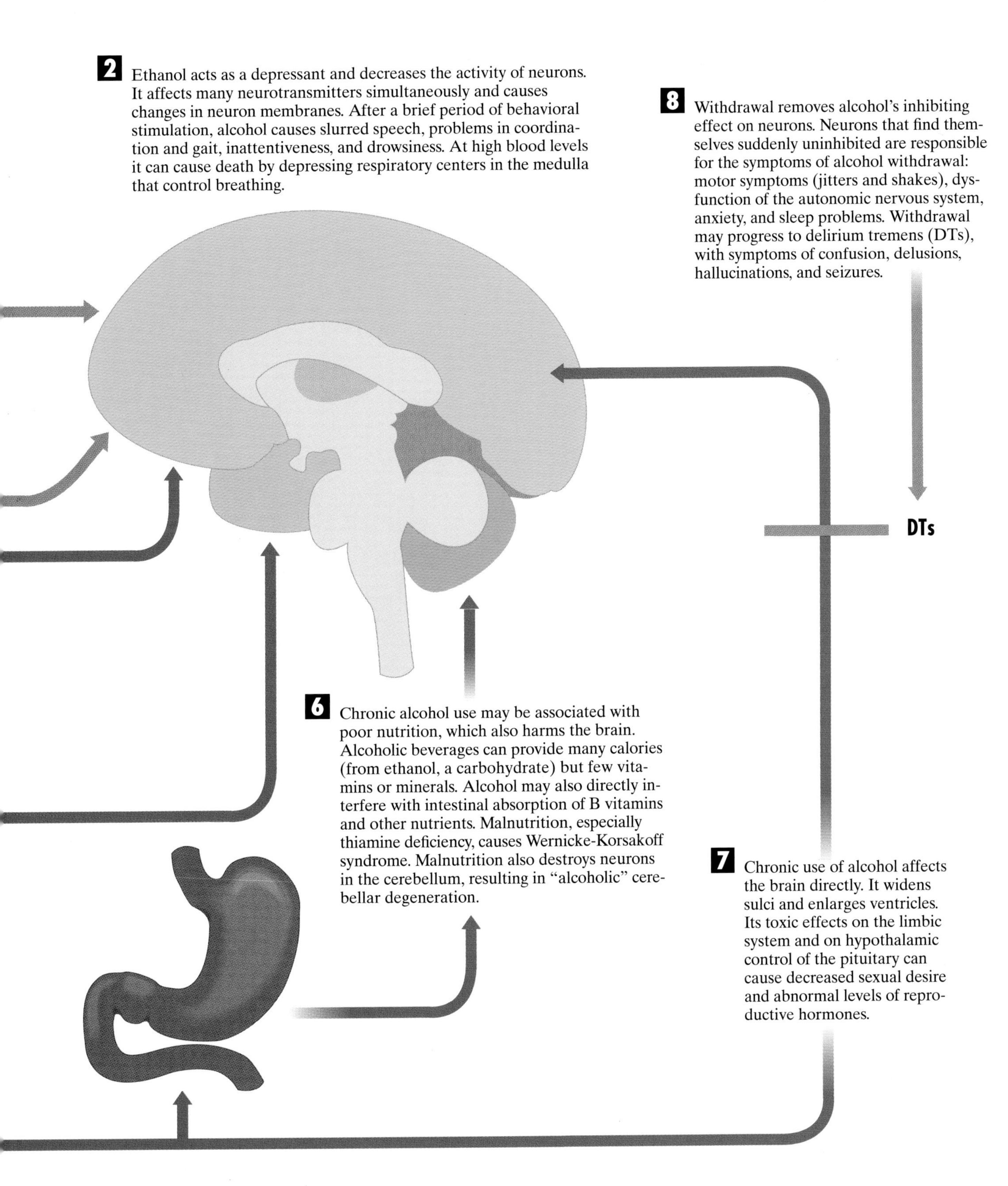
2
Ethanol acts as a depressant and decreases the activity of neurons. It affects many neurotransmitters simultaneously and causes changes in neuron membranes. After a brief period of behavioral stimulation, alcohol causes slurred speech, problems in coordination and gait, inattentiveness, and drowsiness. At high blood levels it can cause death by depressing respiratory centers in the medulla that control breathing.
8
Withdrawal removes alcohol's inhibiting effect on neurons. Neurons that find themselves suddenly uninhibited are responsible for the symptoms of alcohol withdrawal: motor symptoms (jitters and shakes), dysfunction of the autonomic nervous system, anxiety, and sleep problems. Withdrawal may progress to delirium tremens (DTs), with symptoms of confusion, delusions, hallucinations, and seizures.
DTs
6
Chronic alcohol use may be associated with poor nutrition, which also harms the brain. Alcoholic beverages can provide many calories (from ethanol, a carbohydrate) but few vitamins or minerals. Alcohol may also directly interfere with intestinal absorption of B vitamins and other nutrients. Malnutrition, especially thiamine deficiency, causes Wernicke-Korsakoff syndrome. Malnutrition also destroys neurons in the cerebellum, resulting in "alcoholic" cerebellar degeneration.
7
Chronic use of alcohol affects the brain directly. It widens sulci and enlarges ventricles. Its toxic effects on the limbic system and on hypothalamic control of the pituitary can cause decreased sexual desire and abnormal levels of reproductive hormones.

Illegal Drugs: Mechanisms of Environmental Disaster

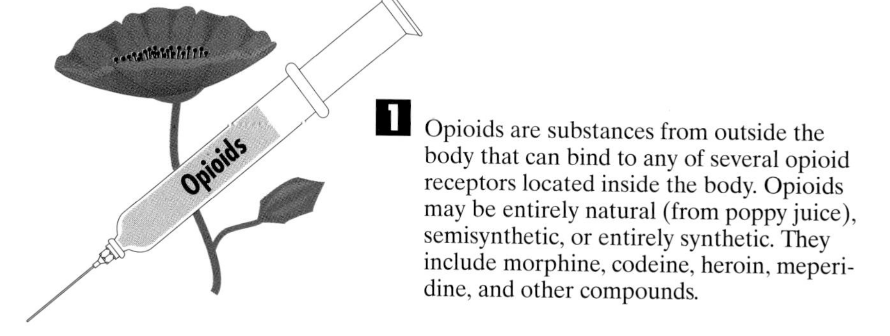

1 Opioids are substances from outside the body that can bind to any of several opioid receptors located inside the body. Opioids may be entirely natural (from poppy juice), semisynthetic, or entirely synthetic. They include morphine, codeine, heroin, meperidine, and other compounds.

2 Different opioids bind to different opioid receptors within the body. Specific types of opioid receptors are identified by specific Greek letters. The "classic" opioids of abuse, such as morphine, may bind preferentially to *mu* receptors. When the body produces its own opioid-like chemicals (enkephalins, endorphins, and others), these seem to bind to other types of opioid receptors.

3 When opioids bind to receptors in the limbic system, they cause euphoria; in the thalamus and spinal cord they decrease pain; and in the medulla they trigger nausea and vomiting. In the hypothalamus and pituitary, opioids cause increased prolactin secretion and decreased secretion of LH and thyrotropin. Overdose of opioids causes unresponsiveness, respiratory depression, decreased heart rate, and constricted pupils. Overdose can cause death from respiratory and cardiac arrest.

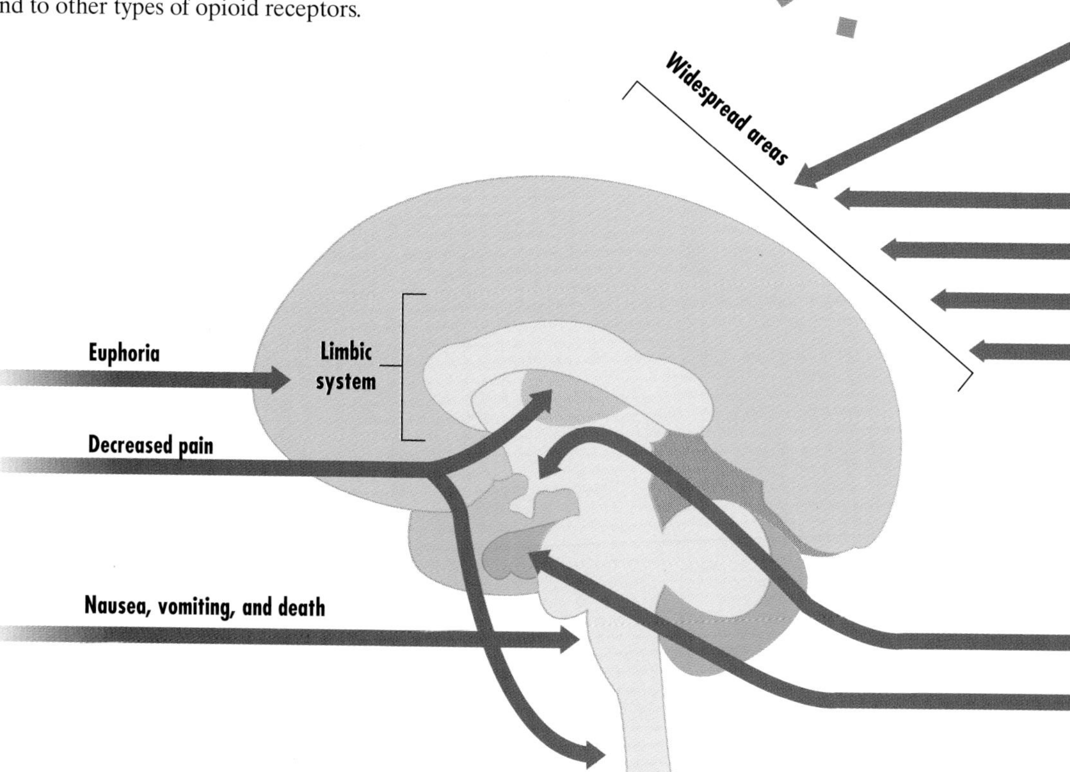

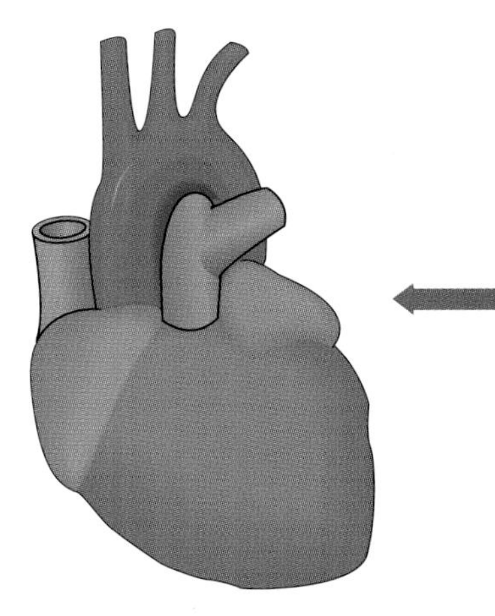

5 High doses of cocaine can cause irregular heartbeat and spasms of the coronary arteries, even a heart attack (myocardial infarction). Cocaine-induced increases in blood pressure can cause brain hemorrhage.

Death

Stimulants

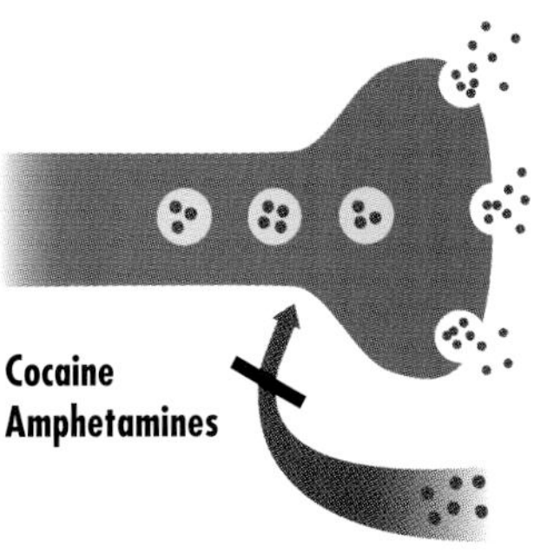

4 Stimulants, like cocaine and the amphetamines, enhance excitation at synapses by blocking the re-uptake of neurotransmitters by neurons. Cocaine blocks re-uptake of dopamine, norepinephrine, and serotonin. Amphetamines definitely block re-uptake of dopamine, and probably block recovery of norepinephrine and serotonin as well. Amphetamines also seem to promote dopamine release.

Euphoria, alertness

Decreased hunger and sleep

Paranoia, suspicion

Hallucinations

6 Cocaine and the amphetamines act on many areas of the brain and on neurons located outside the brain that use norepinephrine as a neurotransmitter. The result is euphoria, increased alertness, decreased hunger, decreased need for sleep, and increased heart rate and blood pressure. There may also be hallucinations of bugs or vermin crawling under the skin, as well as paranoia and suspicion that mimic symptoms of paranoid schizophrenia.

Decreased hormones

Depressed hippocampus

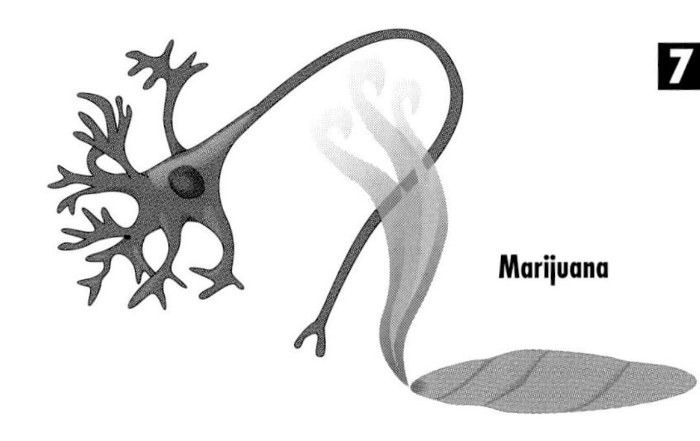

Marijuana

7 Marijuana contains chemicals called cannabinoids. No cannabinoid receptors have been identified in the brain, and marijuana's mechanism of action remains unknown. Marijuana may depress the activity of neurons in the hippocampus, as well as block the hypothalamic releasing hormones ultimately responsible for regulation of the sex hormones. Use of marijuana impairs performance on complex tasks (like driving), elevates mood, and makes time appear to slow down. Chronic use may lead to lack of motivation (amotivational syndrome).

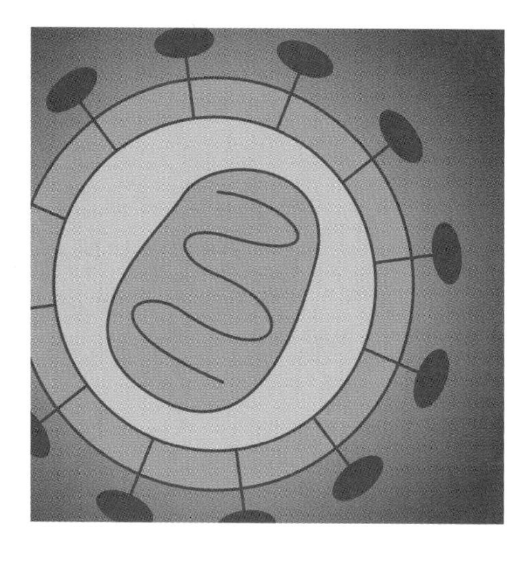

AIDS and the Brain

When Defenses Are Down

ALTHOUGH NEURONS ARE excellent strategists, they are relatively poor warriors. They can not protect themselves. So just as the brain depends on other organs for its energy supply and oxygen, it must rely on the body's immune system for much of its protection against disease. Infection, seen from the perspective of neurons, is a battle between allies and aliens. The allies include lymphocytes and other subtypes of immune cells, while the aliens include viruses, bacteria, and other microscopic life forms that are truly foreign or "alien" to the neural world.

In most types of infection, when alien invaders target a specific body organ for their attack, the immune system responds with its full army of defensive cells to fight off the invasion. In the case of human immunodeficiency virus (HIV) the case is frighteningly different because HIV attacks the ranks of the immune defenders themselves, specifically the T4 lymphocytes.

Once HIV diminishes the number of T4 lymphocytes, the body's depleted immune system becomes less capable of defending against a wide range of infections. And just as a nation without an effective army can be invaded, ravaged, and destroyed from many sides, the body whose defenses are compromised by HIV is at the mercy of many different microscopic enemies. The spectrum of symptoms and illnesses that results when HIV depletes the body's immune defenses forms acquired immune deficiency syndrome, known as AIDS.

At the level of the brain, AIDS begins with an infection by HIV, which has traveled to the brain through the bloodstream and can circulate in the CSF. There is evidence that, once in the brain, the HIV virus may attack certain types of neuroglia directly, just as it directly attacks the T4 lymphocytes of the immune system. Although HIV may not specifically infect neurons, it is probable that toxins and other chemicals produced by HIV can damage neurons and impair neuron function.

HIV infection may cause a wide range of neurologic problems. Within days or weeks of an initial HIV infection, a flu-like illness may develop, with fever, muscle pain, and headache. This illness may progress to meningitis (inflammation of the meninges) and encephalitis (inflammation of the brain).

Chronic HIV infection may impair the brain's more complex neural functions, resulting in AIDS dementia. In AIDS dementia there may be problems in concentration and recall; a slowing of words and actions; and trouble in writing, walking, and performing complex tasks. The mechanism behind these changes may be HIV-induced destruction of white matter and deeper areas of the brain. HIV appears to spare the gray matter.

When HIV compromises the body's immune defenses, the brain is open to attack from other viruses in addition to HIV. Herpes simplex virus (HSV) and cytomegalovirus (CMV), like HIV, can attack the brain and cause meningitis and encephalitis. Another viral agent, the JC virus, is also believed to attack people with HIV infection. The JC virus appears to destroy the white matter of the brain, causing a condition known as progressive multifocal leukoencephalopathy (PML). PML can cause hemiplegia (paralysis of one side of the body), loss of vision, and problems in speaking and in performing other complex mental functions.

In addition to viruses, other aggressive microscopic life forms pose a threat to the HIV-compromised brain. The yeastlike fungus *Cryptococcus neoformans* can cause meningitis in HIV-infected patients, and the protozoan, *Toxoplasma gondii* can cause encephalitis. *Toxoplasma gondii* may also grow within the brain as a mass that is visible on computer tomography (CT) scans.

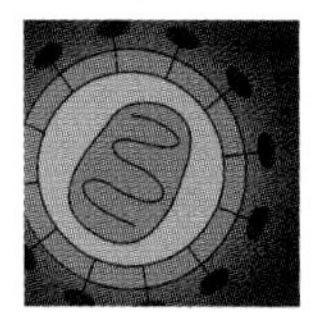

Drugs are available to treat most of the infections associated with HIV. When the infecting agent is CMV, *Toxoplasma*, or *Cryptococcus*, a lifelong program of drug therapy may be necessary.

HIV infection has been associated with a higher risk of primary lymphomas of the brain. These tumors tend to involve multiple sites, especially around the ventricles, within the white matter, and in the subarachnoid space. Treatment with steroids will often shrink lymphomas or make them disappear, but they can recur. Chemotherapy and radiation are also used.

New anti-HIV drugs have the potential to cause problems in the nervous system. Zidovudine (AZT) has side effects that include severe headache, nausea, and insomnia. Both didanosine and zalcitabine can cause peripheral neuropathy, a condition that produces symptoms of tingling, burning, pain, or numbness in the hands and feet.

HIV: Opening the Door to Invaders

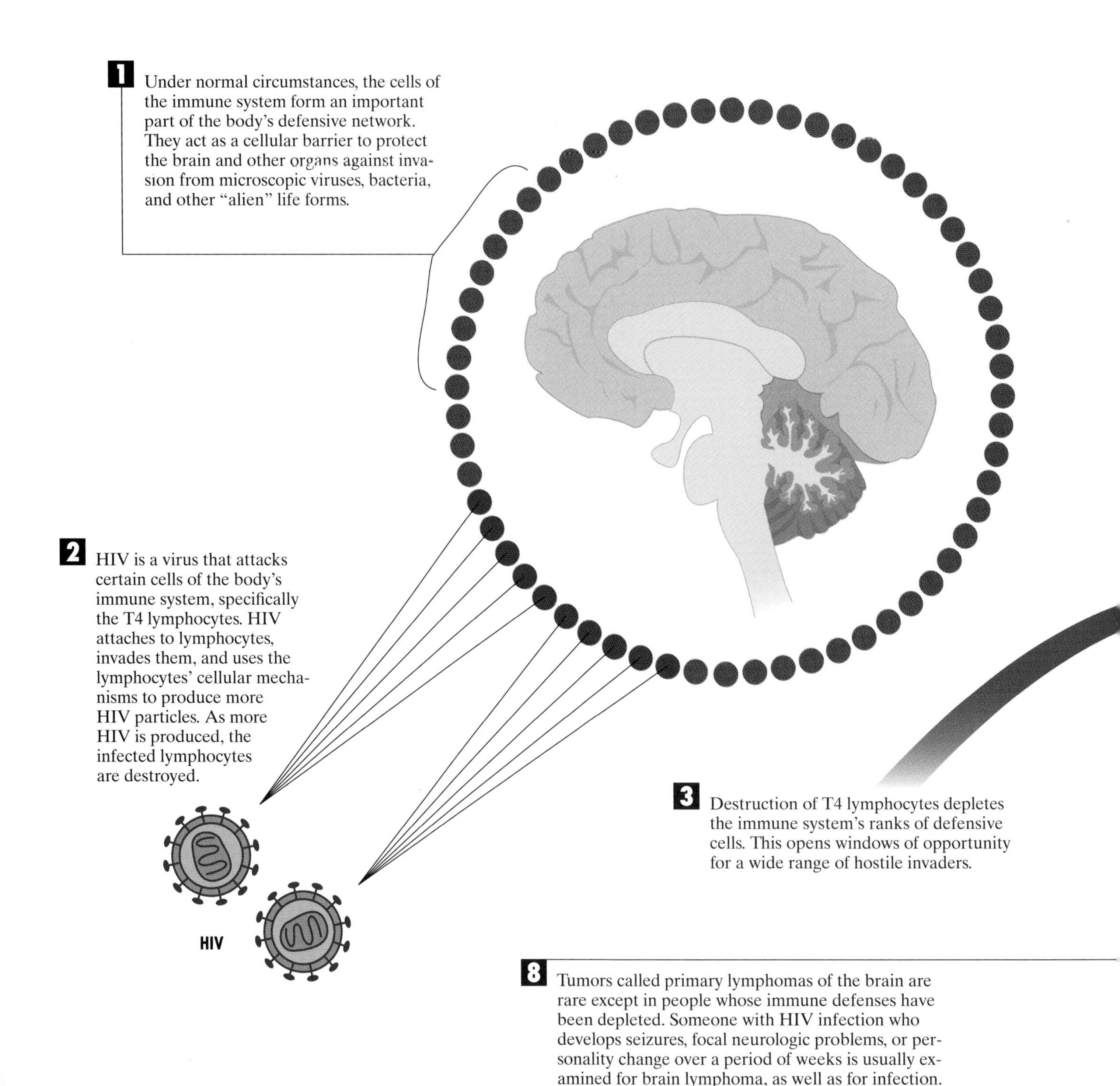

8 Tumors called primary lymphomas of the brain are rare except in people whose immune defenses have been depleted. Someone with HIV infection who develops seizures, focal neurologic problems, or personality change over a period of weeks is usually examined for brain lymphoma, as well as for infection.

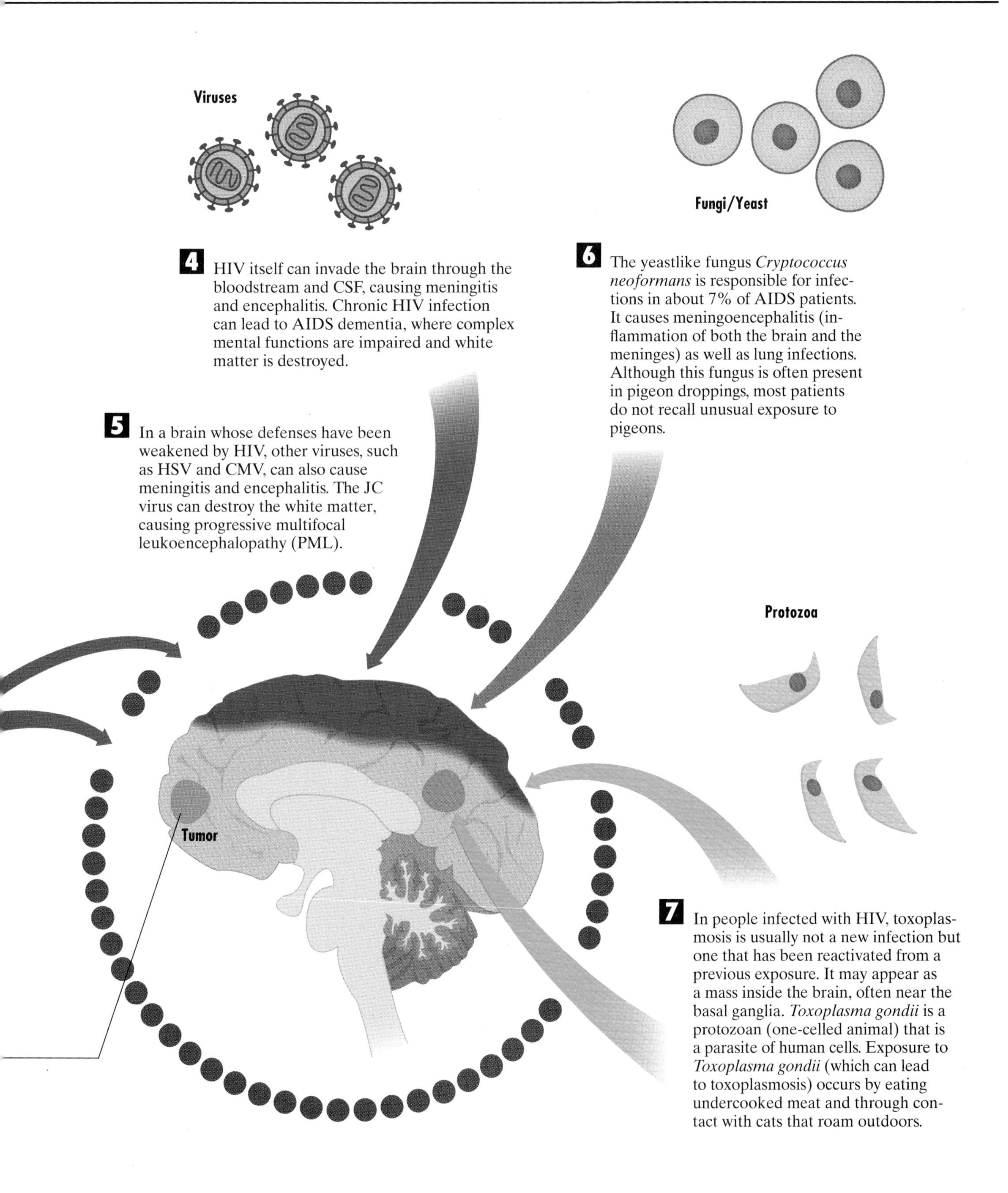

4 HIV itself can invade the brain through the bloodstream and CSF, causing meningitis and encephalitis. Chronic HIV infection can lead to AIDS dementia, where complex mental functions are impaired and white matter is destroyed.

5 In a brain whose defenses have been weakened by HIV, other viruses, such as HSV and CMV, can also cause meningitis and encephalitis. The JC virus can destroy the white matter, causing progressive multifocal leukoencephalopathy (PML).

6 The yeastlike fungus *Cryptococcus neoformans* is responsible for infections in about 7% of AIDS patients. It causes meningoencephalitis (inflammation of both the brain and the meninges) as well as lung infections. Although this fungus is often present in pigeon droppings, most patients do not recall unusual exposure to pigeons.

7 In people infected with HIV, toxoplasmosis is usually not a new infection but one that has been reactivated from a previous exposure. It may appear as a mass inside the brain, often near the basal ganglia. *Toxoplasma gondii* is a protozoan (one-celled animal) that is a parasite of human cells. Exposure to *Toxoplasma gondii* (which can lead to toxoplasmosis) occurs by eating undercooked meat and through contact with cats that roam outdoors.

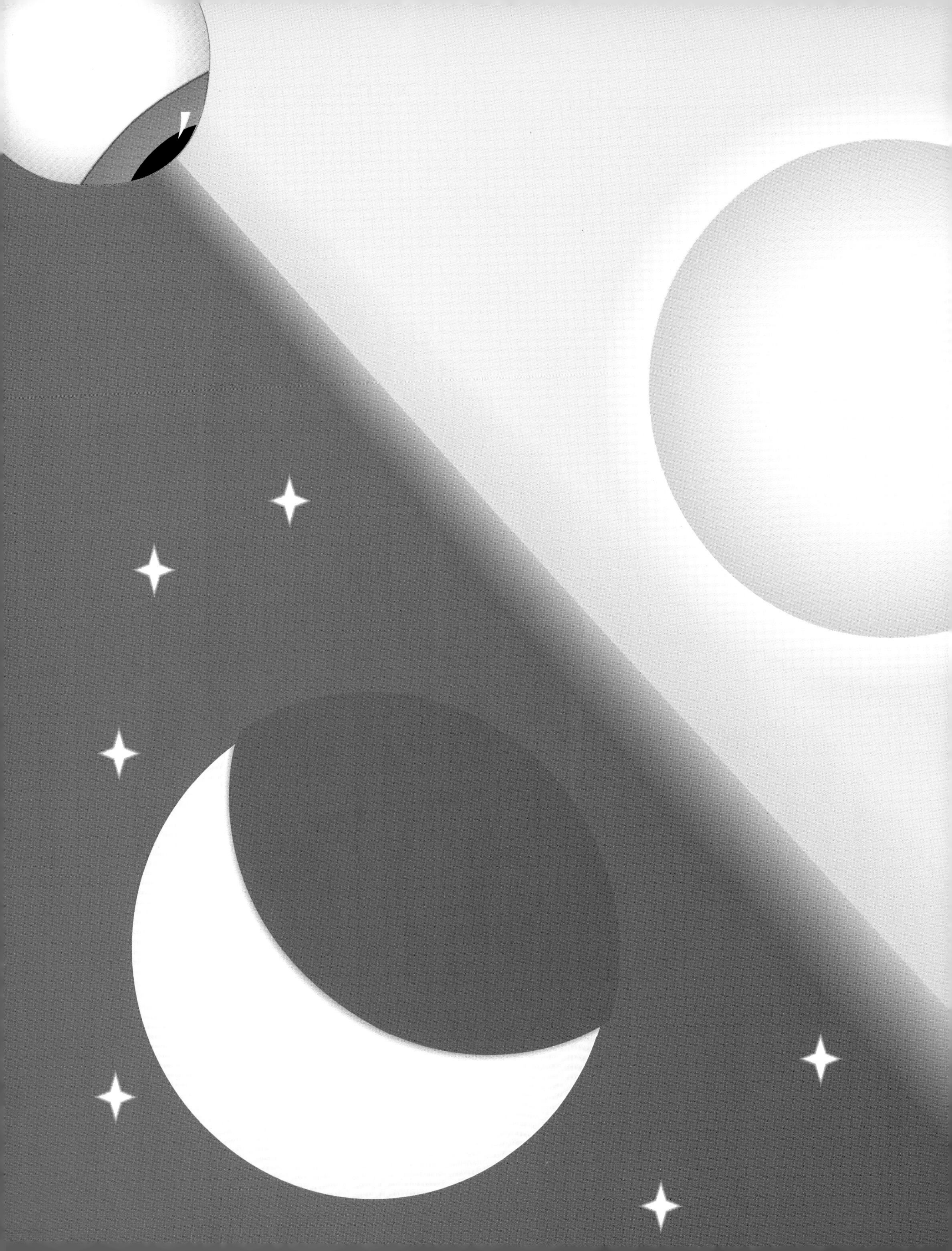

PART

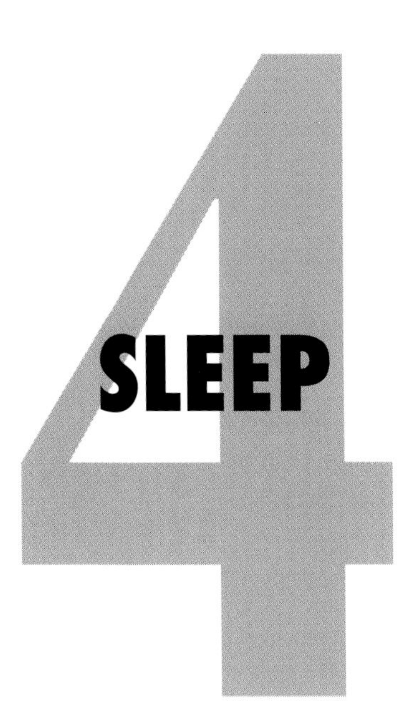

SLEEP

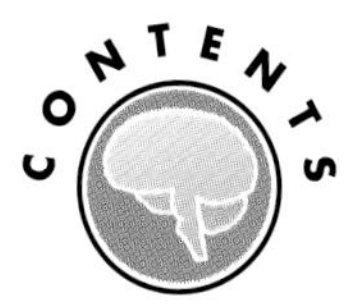

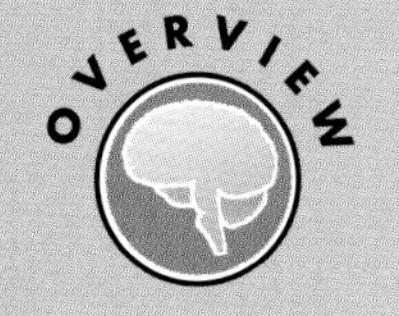
OVERVIEW

IN OUR HUMAN WORLD we have special holidays when we usually leave our work in order to gather with our friends and families. Because we are not performing our everyday jobs, we may appear to be resting, but we are actually very busy. We are busy with hundreds of small rituals that reaffirm our human relationships, renew our strength, and form the substance of our lifetime's memories.

In human terms, sleep is the brain's sustaining ritual. The sleeping brain temporarily stops performing the mundane chores of consciousness in favor of neural activities that appear to renew it and preserve its functional integrity. Without enough sleep, the brain's intellectual activities are sluggish, its emotions are more easily irritated, and its behavior may mimic psychiatric illness.

Yet in spite of the importance of sleep, it remains one of the brain's most secret activities. The unconsciousness of sleep, unlike that of coma, is a fragile state that can be interrupted fairly easily by many different types of outside stimulation. If our scientific studies intrude into the ritual of sleep itself, our measurements and observations may not be correct. And unless we study sleep very delicately, it will disappear before our eyes.

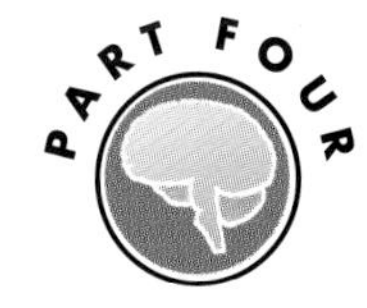

In this book's final pages, we will examine the possible mechanisms behind wakefulness and sleep, and discuss how "sleep factors" may have a role in sleep induction. We will divide the state of sleep into stages based on physiologic changes that occur in different parts of the body, and we will explore what is known about dreams. We will see why the sense of hearing may never truly sleep, and why people who suffer from narcolepsy may not be able to stay awake. We will also examine how the brain's ritual of sleep is disturbed when the body is ill, just as our Thanksgiving dinner might be disturbed in times of war or family tragedy.

The scientific study of sleep is in its infancy, and much is unknown. As a species, we humans have split the atom and walked on the moon before we have understood either the mechanism or the meaning behind our own dreams. And if we ultimately find that our dreams are nothing more than a random firing of neurons, what then? Will this lessen their significance? Or will we find something beyond the synapses that broadens our understanding of our own humanity?

Perhaps the real exploration is just beginning.

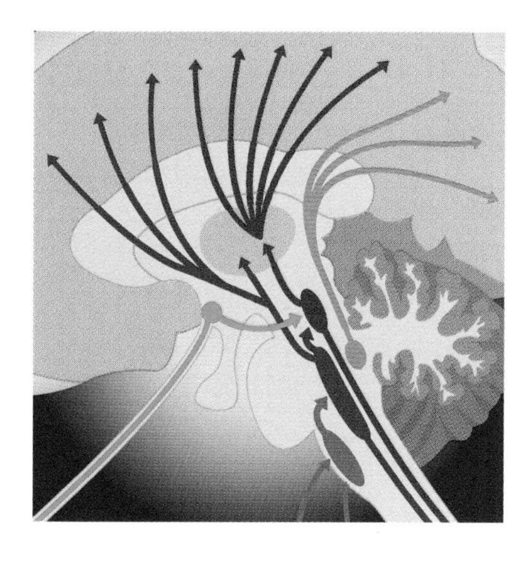

Sleep

Renewing and Sustaining the World

ALTHOUGH THE EXACT REASON for sleep is unknown, the effects of sleep deprivation, including mental sluggishness and irritability, seem to indicate that certain neural systems need a periodic rest from consciousness in order to function properly. Constant wakefulness appears to exhaust certain parts of the brain, and sleep appears to renew them.

In order to properly discuss the mechanisms and effects of sleep, we need to first understand the mechanisms behind wakefulness. Control of wakefulness appears to lie somewhere below the level of the cerebral hemispheres, and current theories place it somewhere in the upper pons. This area, called the *bulboreticular facilitory area*, sends signals for wakefulness to the cerebral hemispheres via pathways that synapse in the thalamus. Many of these pathways use acetylcholine as a neurotransmitter. The cerebral hemisphere's activity (sensory, motor, or higher "thinking" functions) feeds back to the bulboreticular facilitory area and stimulates the brain to even greater wakefulness. So, after the hemispheres are awakened, their own neural activities help to keep them awake. The bulboreticular facilitory area also sends signals down from the pons to the spinal cord to wake up the body's muscles and spinal reflexes. The whole system of neural mechanisms that generates and maintains wakefulness is sometimes called the reticular activating system.

The area responsible for sleep induction appears to be located farther down in the brainstem, in the *raphe nuclei* that lie in the midline of the lower pons and medulla. The raphe nuclei seem to inhibit the brain's wakefulness center, the bulboreticular facilitory area. They also send signals for sleep induction to the thalamus, cerebral cortex, and limbic system, and they send impulses down the spinal cord to inhibit any incoming pain signals from sensory neurons. Because many of the nerve endings of the raphe nuclei secrete serotonin, this particular neurotransmitter is probably the most important inducer of sleep in the brain.

It is possible that many different systems can feed into the sleep induction center to trigger it and cause sleep to begin. Some theorists suggest that prolonged wakefulness causes certain chemicals to accumulate in the body and that these chemicals trigger the raphe nuclei to induce sleep. Some possible sleep-inducing chemicals or "sleep factors" include biochemicals that also have immune activity, suggesting that sleep may be linked to the body's immune defenses. Perhaps the immune system actually signals the brain to sleep as part of a broader mechanism of defense against exhaustion and disease.

Another system for triggering sleep induction comes by way of the ninth (glossopharyngeal) and tenth (vagus) cranial nerves. Signals from either of these nerves appear to excite the sleep induction center and trigger sleep. Our own life experience suggests this connection when we remember how infants tend to fall asleep while nursing (stimulation of the glossopharyngeal nerve), and how humans of all ages tend to feel sleepy after a large meal (stomach distension stimulates the vagus nerve).

Perhaps the most mysterious sleep-inducing input of all comes through pathways from the eyes. The retinohypothalamic tract, a pathway from the retina of the eyes to the hypothalamus, seems to program the suprachiasmatic nuclei of the hypothalamus as light-dark pacemakers. These nuclei may help to synchronize sleep with outside light conditions and may induce sleep by inhibiting the wakefulness center. Because the hypothalamus regulates secretion of so many of the body's hormones, it is also possible that the suprachiasmatic nuclei help coordinate the secretion of several hormones with the passage of day and night.

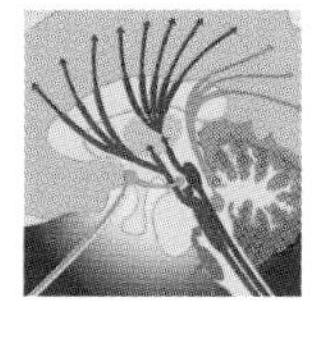

Once sleep has been induced by the raphe nuclei, the conscious activities of the brain are suspended, but a whole new series of unconscious brain activities begins. In order to better study the state of sleep, scientists have divided sleep into two basic patterns, depending on certain physiologic signs. The key sign appears to be rapid movements of the eyes, which are similar to waking eye movements but with the eyelids closed. In *rapid eye movement sleep* or *REM sleep* the body's muscle tone is dramatically decreased (except for the eye muscles), both heart rate and breathing are irregular, and abnormal heart rhythms may occur. The body temporarily loses its ability to regulate body temperature, and becomes transiently cold-blooded. This is usually not a problem, however, since extreme temperatures also seem to prevent REM sleep. During periods of REM sleep, the brain is very active, its metabolism may increase up to 20%, and its brain wave pattern is similar to wakefulness. We have dreams during REM sleep and we tend to remember them.

In *non-REM sleep* or *NREM sleep*, there are no rapid eye movements, and although we may also dream during NREM sleep, the dreams are less vivid and less likely to be remembered. During NREM sleep the body's metabolism decreases, breathing slows, and the blood pressure usually drops by 10% to 20%. NREM sleep may be especially restful for the brain, since the brain seems to need greater amounts of NREM sleep than REM sleep after long periods of sleep deprivation.

During the night, periods of NREM sleep are followed by REM sleep, forming a NREM-REM sleep cycle that repeats about every 90 to 110 minutes. Each REM episode accounts for 5 to 30 minutes of each NREM-REM cycle, and a person typically awakens in the morning during an episode of REM sleep.

Although we do not know why the brain has NREM-REM cycles, it is believed that a center in the locus ceruleus of the pons regulates REM sleep through fibers that use the neurotransmitter norepinephrine. How this center can stimulate and activate many different brain areas without awakening the brain to consciousness is also unknown.

Although the sleeping brain is not conscious, it remains unconsciously aware of selected types of stimulation. Loud sounds, for example, are especially effective sleep eliminators, and this is the reason why alarm clocks work so well. The pathways responsible for this are collateral fibers from the auditory tracts (Chapter 7). Auditory signals from loud sounds pass down these collaterals directly into the wakefulness center, which activates the entire brain and spinal cord.

Sleep abnormalities can interfere with waking activities. People who suffer from narcolepsy, for example, often feel sleepy during their waking hours and complain of disturbed sleep at night. They have involuntary episodes of sleep during the daytime and may have episodes of sudden weakness or loss of muscle tone (cataplexy). Narcolepsy appears to be a hereditary condition that is related to abnormalities in REM sleep. Its symptoms are treated with medications.

Daytime sleepiness may also be caused by various types of breathing problems that occur during sleep. In the sleep apnea syndromes, breathing stops for periods that last anywhere from 15 seconds to over 2 minutes. This happens either because the airways are blocked by relaxed throat muscles or because the brain's regulatory mechanisms for breathing are not functioning properly. Episodes of sleep apnea lead to decreased oxygen and increased carbon dioxide in the blood. This results in physiologic changes in the brain and elsewhere that have been implicated as causes of memory loss, personality disturbances, impotence, hypertension, heart and lung disorders, and unexplained death during sleep.

Sleep may be disturbed by medical and neuropsychiatric illnesses. People who suffer from depression often sleep poorly and have been found to have disturbances in both REM and NREM sleep. Cluster headaches are characteristically related to sleep, although the mechanism is unknown. People with angina may experience nightmares or chest pain during sleep, because of changes in the heart and blood vessels that occur during REM sleep episodes.

And, finally, what do we know about dreams? We know that while dreams occur in both NREM and REM sleep, those in REM sleep are more vivid and memorable. We also know that our dreams can be influenced by sensations (hunger, thirst, pain) and by thoughts, ideas, and feelings that are carried over from our waking lives.

How can we explain the content of dreams in terms of neural pathways? Interestingly, recent theories that link anxiety and the digestive system also involve the locus ceruleus (Chapter 14), and we have seen that the locus ceruleus controls REM sleep. Maybe we will soon find that digestive upset can influence our REM dreams by way of the locus ceruleus. If so, it might be comforting to know that at least some of our nightmares, as Dickens's Scrooge suggested, have more to do with gravy than with graves.

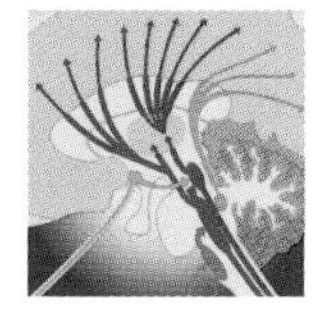

As for more complex Freudian theories, we have much more to learn about the brain before we can hope to relate these elaborate explanations to actual pathways in the neural world.

The World Wakes and Sleeps: Central Regulation

6 Certain biochemical "sleep factors" may accumulate when the brain and body have been awake for long periods. They may circulate in the blood and CSF and act directly on the brain to induce sleep.

5 The retinohypothalamic tract brings information about light-dark cycles to the suprachiasmatic nuclei of the hypothalamus. These nuclei probably help to coordinate sleep with light-dark cycles (circadian rhythms). They may also help to induce sleep by inhibiting the wakefulness center when night falls.

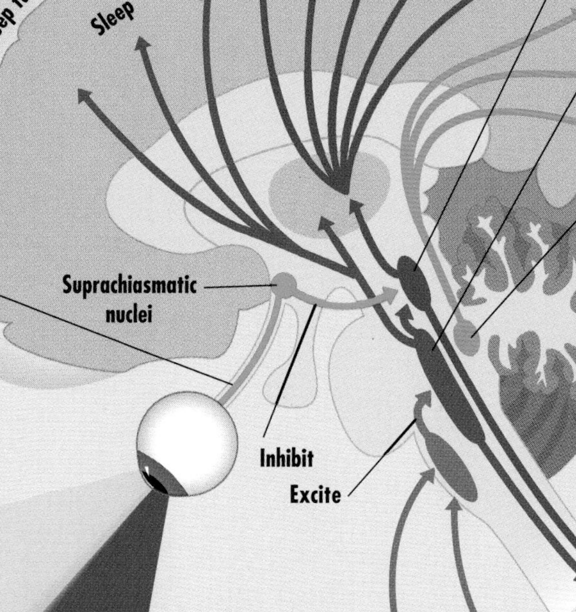

1 Wakefulness (shown here as red pathways) is probably controlled by a facilitory center in the upper pons. This center sends signals to the cerebral cortex through excitatory pathways that synapse in the thalamus. Awakening impulses also travel down the spinal cord.

2 Sleep is probably induced by the raphe nuclei of the lower pons and medulla. These nuclei send inhibitory impulses (shown here as blue) to the facilitory center as well as to the cortex, limbic system, and thalamus. Their inhibitory impulses to the spinal cord also block incoming pain sensation.

3 Sleep is divided into REM and NREM periods (see preceding pages). REM sleep, associated with vivid dreams, may be controlled by the locus ceruleus, a nucleus in the pons. The locus sends impulses to excite many areas of the cortex without awakening the brain to consciousness.

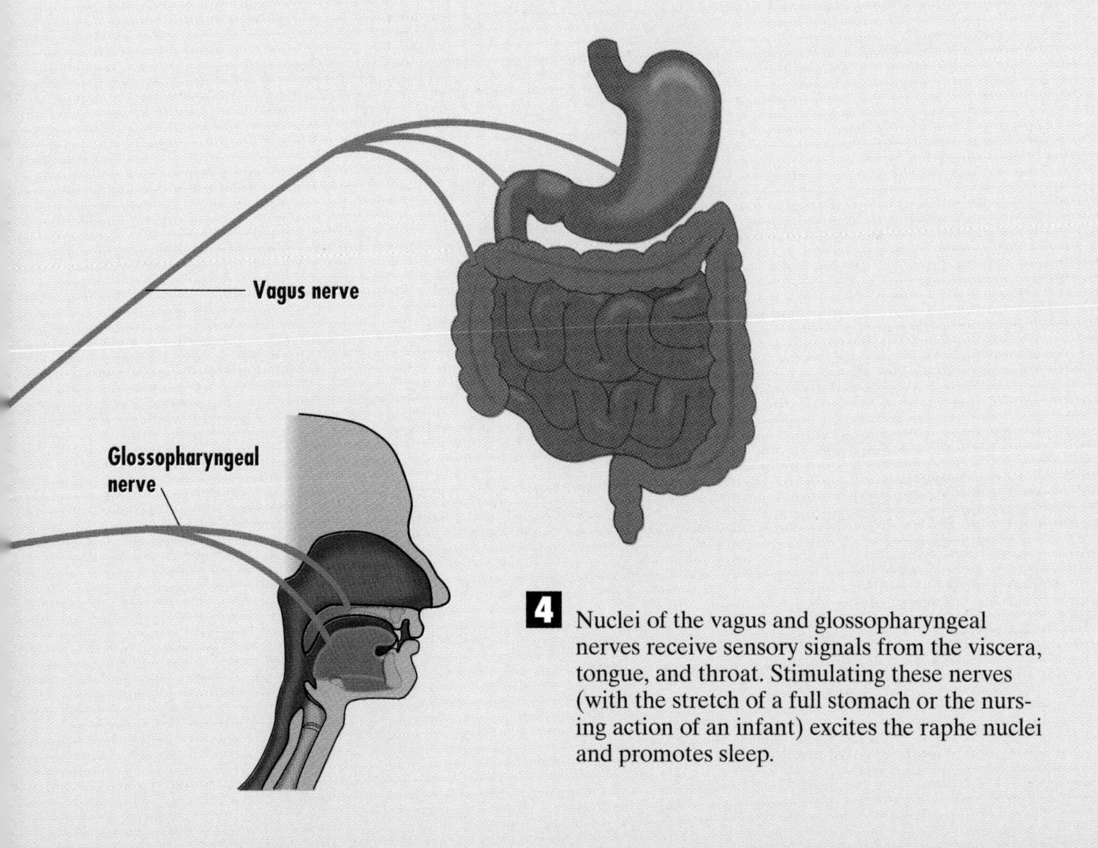

4 Nuclei of the vagus and glossopharyngeal nerves receive sensory signals from the viscera, tongue, and throat. Stimulating these nerves (with the stretch of a full stomach or the nursing action of an infant) excites the raphe nuclei and promotes sleep.

A

V

W

Z